Specialty Competencies in Rehabilitation Psychology

Series in Specialty Competencies in Professional Psychology

SERIES EDITORS

Arthur M. Nezu, PhD, ABPP, and Christine Maguth Nezu, PhD, ABPP

SERIES ADVISORY BOARD

David Barlow, PhD, ABPP

Jon Carlson, PsyD, EdD, ABPP

Kirk Heilbrun, PhD, ABPP

Nadine J. Kaslow, PhD, ABPP

Robert Klepac, PhD

William Parham, PhD, ABPP

Michael G. Perri, PhD, ABPP

C. Steven Richards, PhD

Norma P. Simon, EdD, ABPP

TITLES IN THE SERIES

Specialty Competencies in School Psychology, Rosemary Flanagan and Jeffrey A. Miller

Specialty Competencies in Organizational and Business Consulting Psychology, Jay C. Thomas

Specialty Competencies in Geropsychology, Victor Molinari (Ed.)

Specialty Competencies in Forensic Psychology, Ira K. Packer and Thomas Grisso

Specialty Competencies in Couple and Family Psychology, Mark Stanton and Robert Welsh

Specialty Competencies in Clinical Child and Adolescent Psychology, Alfred J. Finch, Jr., John E. Lochman, W. Michael Nelson III, and Michael C. Roberts

Specialty Competencies in Clinical Neuropsychology, Greg J. Lamberty and Nathaniel W. Nelson

Specialty Competencies in Counseling Psychology, Jairo N. Fuertes, Arnold Spokane, and Elizabeth Holloway

Specialty Competencies in Group Psychology, Sally Barlow

Specialty Competencies in Clinical Psychology, Robert A. DiTomasso, Stacey C. Cahn, Susan M. Panichelli-Mindel, and Roger K. McFillin

Specialty Competencies in Rehabilitation Psychology, David R. Cox, Richard H. Cox, and Bruce Caplan

DAVID R. COX
RICHARD H. COX
BRUCE CAPLAN

Specialty Competencies in Rehabilitation Psychology

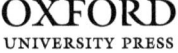

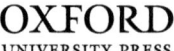

Oxford University Press is a department of the University of Oxford.
It furthers the University's objective of excellence in research, scholarship,
and education by publishing worldwide.

Oxford   New York
Auckland   Cape Town   Dar es Salaam   Hong Kong   Karachi
Kuala Lumpur   Madrid   Melbourne   Mexico City   Nairobi
New Delhi   Shanghai   Taipei   Toronto

With offices in
Argentina   Austria   Brazil   Chile   Czech Republic   France   Greece
Guatemala   Hungary   Italy   Japan   Poland   Portugal   Singapore
South Korea   Switzerland   Thailand   Turkey   Ukraine   Vietnam

Oxford is a registered trademark of Oxford University Press in the UK and certain other
countries.

Published in the United States of America by
Oxford University Press
198 Madison Avenue, New York, NY 10016

© Oxford University Press 2013

All rights reserved. No part of this publication may be reproduced, stored in a
retrieval system, or transmitted, in any form or by any means, without the prior
permission in writing of Oxford University Press, or as expressly permitted by law,
by license, or under terms agreed with the appropriate reproduction rights organization.
Inquiries concerning reproduction outside the scope of the above should be sent to the Rights
Department, Oxford University Press, at the address above.

You must not circulate this work in any other form
and you must impose this same condition on any acquirer.

Library of Congress Cataloging-in-Publication Data
Cox, David R.
Specialty competencies in rehabilitation psychology / David R. Cox, Richard H. Cox, Bruce Caplan.
    pages cm.—(Series in specialty competencies in professional psychology)
Includes bibliographical references and index.
ISBN 978-0-19-538924-1 (pbk.)
1. Clinical psychology.   2. Core competencies.   3. Psychotherapists—Training of.
I. Cox, Richard H.   II. Caplan, Bruce.   III. Title.
RC467.C685 2014
616.89—dc23
2013023208

SELECTED EVENTS IN THE HISTORY OF REHABILITATION PSYCHOLOGY

1940s–1950s	Psychologists became increasingly involved in caring for persons with disabilities, many resulting from battlefield injury in World War II.
1949	The National Council on Psychological Aspects of Disability (NCPAD) established.
1951	NCPAD formally affiliated with American Psychological Association (APA) as a special interest group.
1955	NCPAD voted to seek division status within the APA.
1956	Publication of "Adjustment to Misfortune—A Problem of Social Psychological Rehabilitation" (Dembo, Leviton, & Wright).
1958	Establishment of Division of Rehabilitation Psychology (Division 22) of APA.
1958 and 1959	Office of Vocational Rehabilitation in the Department of Health, Education and Welfare helped sponsor conferences whose purpose was defining rehabilitation psychology.
1958	The Princeton Conference was held in February of 1958 and was also sponsored by the APA.
1959	Publication of Beatrice Wright's book, *Psychology and Rehabilitation*, a product of the Princeton Conference proceedings.
1959	Clark University Conference focused on increased research in the field of rehabilitation psychology as well as a need for suitable vehicles for publication of such research. *Rehabilitation Psychology*, the official journal of Division 22, emerged from this process, having initially begun as *The Bulletin*.
1960	Beatrice Wright's seminal *Physical Disability: A Psychosocial Approach* published.
1962	Publication of *Psychological Practices With the Physically Disabled* (Garrett & Levine).
1970	National Conference on the Psychological Aspects of Disability, Monterey, CA.
1971	Publication of *Rehabilitation Psychology* (Neff), based on papers from the Monterey Conference.
1970s–1980s	Growth in the area of neurorehabilitation led to a marked increase in the number of rehabilitation psychologists treating persons with brain injury and other neurological disorders.
1980	Publication of *Spinal Cord Injuries: Psychological, Social and Vocational Adjustment* (Trieschmann).

1987	Publication of *Rehabilitation Psychology Desk Reference* (Caplan).
Early 1990s	Led by the Division of Rehabilitation Psychology, the field began to explore whether a desire and/or need existed to more clearly delineate rehabilitation psychology as a specialty area and *rehabilitation psychologists* as specialists. A specialty credentialing committee was established to review this area and make recommendations.
1995	Publication of *Postdoctoral Training Guidelines for Rehabilitation Psychology* (Patterson & Hanson).
1995	Establishment of the American Board of Rehabilitation Psychology (ABRP).
1995	Division 22 voted to support the ABRP application to the American Board of Professional Psychology (ABPP) for affiliation as a specialty area.
1997	The ABRP became affiliated with the ABPP, with the first group of rehabilitation psychologists being granted ABPP board certification in 1997.
1999	The ABRP and Division 22 joined forces to establish a conference specifically oriented toward education and opportunities for collegial interaction among rehabilitation psychologists.
1999	*Rehabilitation Psychology* journal acquired by Educational Publishing Foundation (subsidiary of the APA).
2000	Publication of *Handbook of Rehabilitation Psychology* (Frank & Elliott).
2006	*Rehabilitation Psychology* journal became an official publication of the APA.
2008	Division 22 awarded the Lifetime Practice Excellence Award to the founding members of the ABRP in honor of their efforts and achievements.
2010	Second edition of *Handbook of Rehabilitation Psychology* (Frank, Rosenthal, & Caplan) published.
2011	The Baltimore Conference on Rehabilitation Psychology Postdoctoral Training was held and developed consensus guidelines on how postdoctoral training programs in rehabilitation psychology should be conducted and the competencies that should be developed, and created the structure for a national organization of postdoctoral training programs in rehabilitation psychology.
2012	The Council of Rehabilitation Psychology Postdoctoral Training Programs initial meeting at the Rehabilitation Psychology conference in February of 2012.

CONTENTS

	About the Series in Specialty Competencies in Professional Psychology	ix
	Preface	xiii

PART I	**Introduction to Rehabilitation Psychology**	
ONE	Introduction: A Brief History of Rehabilitation Psychology	3

PART II	**Foundational Competencies**	
TWO	Ethical and Legal Issues	15
THREE	Individual and Cultural Diversity	31
FOUR	Interpersonal Interaction	41
FIVE	Professional Identity	49

PART III	**Functional Competencies**	
SIX	Assessment	59
SEVEN	Consultation	81
EIGHT	Consumer Protection	101
NINE	Intervention	107
TEN	Science Base and Knowledge	123
ELEVEN	Supervision, Teaching, and Management	143

	References	149
	Key Terms	173

Index	179
About the Authors	189
About the Series Editors	193

ABOUT THE SERIES IN SPECIALTY COMPETENCIES IN PROFESSIONAL PSYCHOLOGY

This series is intended to describe state-of-the-art functional and foundational competencies in professional psychology across extant and emerging specialty areas. Each book in this series provides a guide to best practices across both core and specialty competencies as defined by a given professional psychology specialty.

The impetus for this series was created by various growing movements in professional psychology during the past 15 years. First, as an applied discipline, psychology is increasingly recognizing the unique and distinct nature among a variety of orientations, modalities, and approaches with regard to professional practice. These specialty areas represent distinct ways of practicing one's profession across various domains of activities that are based on distinct bodies of literature and often address differing populations or problems. For example, the American Psychological Association (APA) in 1995 established the Commission on the Recognition of Specialties and Proficiencies in Professional Psychology (CRSPPP) in order to define criteria by which a given specialty could be recognized. The Council of Credentialing Organizations in Professional Psychology (CCOPP), an interorganizational entity, was formed in reaction to the need to establish criteria and principles regarding the types of training programs related to the education, training, and professional development of individuals seeking such specialization. In addition, the Council on Specialties in Professional Psychology (COS) was formed in 1997, independent of the APA, to foster communication among the established specialties, in order to offer a unified position to the pubic regarding specialty education and training, credentialing, and practice standards across specialty areas.

Simultaneously, efforts to actually define professional competence regarding psychological practice have also been growing significantly. For example, the APA-sponsored Task Force on Assessment of Competence in Professional

Psychology put forth a series of guiding principles for the assessment of competence within professional psychology, based, in part, on a review of competency assessment models developed both within (e.g., Assessment of Competence Workgroup from Competencies Conference—Roberts et al., 2005) and outside (e.g., Accreditation Council for Graduate Medical Education and American Board of Medical Specialties, 2000) the profession of psychology (Kaslow et al., 2007).

Moreover, additional professional organizations in psychology have provided valuable input into this discussion, including various associations primarily interested in the credentialing of professional psychologists, such as the American Board of Professional Psychology (ABPP), the Association of State and Provincial Psychology Boards (ASPBB), and the National Register of Health Service Providers in Psychology. This widespread interest and importance of the issue of competency in professional psychology can be especially appreciated given the attention and collaboration afforded to this effort by international groups, including the Canadian Psychological Association and the International Congress on Licensure, Certification, and Credentialing in Professional Psychology.

Each volume in the series is devoted to a specific specialty and provides a definition, description, and development timeline of that specialty, including its essential and characteristic pattern of activities, as well as its distinctive and unique features. Each set of authors, long-term experts and veterans of a given specialty, were asked to describe that specialty along the lines of both functional and foundational competencies. *Functional competencies* are those common practice activities provided at the specialty level of practice that include, for example, the application of its science base, assessment, intervention, consultation, and, where relevant, supervision, management, and teaching. *Foundational competencies* represent core knowledge areas that are integrated and cut across all functional competencies to varying degrees, and dependent upon the specialty, in various ways. These include ethical and legal issues, individual and cultural diversity considerations, interpersonal interactions, and professional identification.

Although we realize that each specialty is likely to undergo changes in the future, we wanted to establish a baseline of basic knowledge and principles that compose a specialty, highlighting both its commonalities with other areas of professional psychology and its distinctiveness. We look forward to seeing the dynamics of such changes, as well as the emergence of new specialties in the future.

In this volume, Drs. Cox, Cox, and Caplan provide an impressive contribution to the series through a comprehensive presentation of the competencies focused on the specialty of rehabilitation psychology. This exceptionally well-written volume reveals the unique contributions of rehabilitation psychology and illustrates the wide range of interrelated issues that are confronted by the rehabilitation specialist on a daily basis. Psychologists and trainees who have an interest in specializing in rehabilitation settings would be well served to use this volume as their "go to" resource for tackling the challenging issues inherent in assisting persons with disabilities to actualize satisfying and meaningful lives. The insights of these experienced rehabilitation specialists are remarkable. Of particular value is the clear and succinct style with which they delineate the wide range of assessment and treatment considerations that need to be integrated as an essential art of competent practice. These include, but are not limited to, considerations concerning the causes of injury and disability, family factors, medical factors, legal factors, and neuropsychological and personality testing.

Arthur M. Nezu
Christine Maguth Nezu

PREFACE

Rehabilitation psychology has undergone impressive growth in recent years, as indicated by, among other things, the development of education and training guidelines and establishment as a recognized specialty under the auspices of the American Board of Rehabilitation Psychology. The authors of the present volume were among the founding members of the American Board of Rehabilitation Psychology, which, as of this writing, has board-certified 149 specialists.

Because formal training programs in rehabilitation psychology are still relatively few in number, many psychologists working in rehabilitation settings arrive there having completed training in related specialties such as clinical psychology, health psychology, neuropsychology, or educational psychology. For such individuals, this volume may serve as a portal to the principles and practices of the specialty. For those seeking board certification, the book may serve as part review and part tutorial, with the caveat that the field continues to evolve and preparation for the board certification process will require familiarity with the latest literature.

It should be noted that the present volume focuses on rehabilitation psychology as it is practiced in the United States. However, practitioners in other countries such as England, Russia, Israel, Australia, New Zealand, and Germany have made substantive contributions as well. Indeed, we would be remiss if we did not recognize the writings of individuals such as Kurt Goldstein (1942), Alexander Luria (1963), and Oliver Zangwill (1947), who did pioneering work in rehabilitation psychology, albeit largely in isolation, and whose work merits rediscovery by each new generation of rehabilitation psychologists.

PART I

Introduction to Rehabilitation Psychology

ONE

Introduction

A Brief History of Rehabilitation Psychology

The "Adam" of rehabilitation psychology is difficult to identify, although the organizational roots are more readily discerned. Larson and Sachs (2000) cite efforts of churches and other charitable organizations during the Middle Ages that could be viewed as precursors of rehabilitation psychology. Meyerson (1963), referring to similar activities, alludes to work of a rehabilitation psychology nature in the 1700s. There is no clear record of these early works and, of course, the field of psychology itself was not yet officially established. Rather, it has largely been since the 1940s that rehabilitation psychology as we now know it has evolved. Detailed review of the history of rehabilitation psychology can be found in the citations referenced in this chapter; the current effort aims to provide an overview.

Contemporary rehabilitation psychology is widely considered to have begun to crystallize during the 1940s and 1950s, as psychologists became increasingly involved in caring for persons with disabilities, many resulting from battlefield injury. While some early rehabilitation psychologists worked independently, many labored within organizations such as the Red Cross, the Easter Seal Society, and the Veterans Administration (now the Department of Veterans Affairs). Government efforts to return injured workers to productivity led to the legislation and establishment of departments focused on vocational rehabilitation; as a result of this, the activity of early rehabilitation psychology practitioners had a significant vocational emphasis.

In a lengthy disquisition that could be viewed as the first major rehabilitation psychology publication, Dembo, Leviton, and Wright (1956) reported on a study of 177 individuals with disabilities, more than half with amputations. Their monograph addressed the issue embodied in the title ("Adjustment to misfortune") as well as outlining the social-psychological underpinnings of much of the early work in the field.

Three other landmark publications of great historical significance should be mentioned. Beatrice Wright's *Physical disability: A psychological approach* (1960; second edition, 1983) is an enduring classic that expanded discussion of many central principles of the specialty including the role of value change in coming to terms with acquired disability, the impact of societal attitudes toward persons with disabilities, and the central role of the patient as a "comanager" of their rehabilitation. In the revised edition, Wright described "20 value-laden beliefs" that encapsulated core principles of her clinical work; 30 years later, these notions still offer an excellent framework for the practicing clinician.

A 1962 volume edited by Garrett and Levine consisted of a dozen chapters, each describing a disabling condition (e.g., cerebral palsy, hemiplegia, sensory disability) that could benefit from psychological assessment and intervention. A 1970 conference in Monterey, California sponsored by APA and the United States Department of Health, Education and Welfare yielded an edited volume (Neff, 1971) with contributions by several early shapers of the field including Leonard Diller, Wilbert Fordyce, and Franklin Shontz.

James Garrett, a founder of the American Psychological Association (APA) Division 22 and associate director of the Office of Vocational Rehabilitation in the Department of Health, Education and Welfare, helped sponsor conferences whose purpose was to define rehabilitation psychology (Larson and Sachs, 2000; Wright, 1959); Victor Raimy served as chairman of the Planning Committee. Two major conferences were held, one at Princeton University in Princeton, New Jersey (subsequently known as the Princeton Conference), and another at Clark University in Worcester, Massachusetts.

The Princeton Conference in February of 1958 was also sponsored by the APA, which published Wright's (1959) book, *Psychology and Rehabilitation*, a product of the conference proceedings.

A consensus about the definition of rehabilitation psychology proved difficult, if not impossible, to obtain. There was broad agreement among those involved in the early definitional efforts about certain distinctive features of rehabilitation psychology such as the emphasis in assessment on measuring not only an individual's deficits but also his or her strengths; providing person-centered treatment aimed toward accommodation/

adaptation and/or restoration of function; a view of injury prevention as a fundamental construct; and a multifactorial perspective on "disability" that views the person with a disability as interacting with and affected by multiple aspects of his or her environment (Wright, 1959). Thus, rehabilitation psychology can claim to have originated the widely accepted biopsychosocial perspective on behavior some two decades before Engel's (1977) classic paper suggesting the term.

At the time of these conferences, there was some discussion about establishing a specialty of rehabilitation psychology; however, "In the interest of furthering the alliance between psychology and rehabilitation, the creation of a new specialty, 'rehabilitation psychology,' was considered and rejected for the present" (Wright, 1959, p. 88). This rejection was primarily with reference to specialization within doctoral psychology training. There was recognition that broad psychological education, training, and experience were necessary for all psychologists, that various areas of psychology could contribute to rehabilitation, and that rehabilitation psychology had much to offer the rest of psychology. It was generally agreed that specialization could, perhaps, occur more optimally following doctoral training. The conference attendees desired to deepen the relation between psychology and rehabilitation and felt that more flexible recommendations allowed for a greater likelihood of evolution of the field. Meyerson (1963, pp. 45–46) would reiterate the notion that given the relative youth of the field, formalization and establishment of "...rigid curriculum for the training of the people who do it..." would be a mistake. Referencing various areas of psychology, he stated, "It draws from all of these and others, and gives something of its own to all of them."

The 1959 Clark University Conference focused on increasing research in the field of rehabilitation psychology as well as a need for suitable vehicles for publication of such research. *Rehabilitation Psychology*, the official journal of Division 22, emerged from this process (Larson and Sachs, 2000), having begun as *The Bulletin* (Brownsberger, 2004).

A vital product of the conferences at Princeton and Clark was a growing interest in formalizing interactions of those involved. Although independent from the aforementioned conferences, some of those in attendance played central roles in facilitating organizational structure for the field.

Evolution of an American Psychological Association Division

Concerted efforts over nearly a decade eventually led to the formation of what is now the Division of Rehabilitation Psychology (APA Division 22) in 1958 (Wright, 1993). The National Council on Psychological Aspects of Disability (NCPAD), helped establish in 1949, formally affiliated with APA in 1951 as a special interest group. The NCPAD became the National Council on Psychological Aspects of Physical Disability (NCPAPD) in 1952 and reverted to NCPAD in name in 1956 (Larson and Sachs, 2000).

According to Larson and Sachs (2000), the membership of the NCPAD initially voted against applying to become a division of the APA. However, that sentiment changed sufficiently such that a petition was put forth in the fall of 1955 with 155 of the 180 members seeking division status. In August 1958, the APA Council of Representatives voted to grant division status to the 22nd division of the APA. Until 1963, the division remained the NCPAD; from 1963 to 1972 it was known as the Division on Psychological Aspects of Disability (DPAD) and has since been the Division of Rehabilitation Psychology. In the first few years, the division grew to a membership of almost 1,000 (Meyerson, 1963); as of this writing, membership stands at about 1,200.

The Division of Rehabilitation Psychology is now over 50 years old. It is a vibrant division and has grown to include formal sections and/or special interest groups such as pediatric rehabilitation, women's issues in rehabilitation, outcomes measurement, assistive technology, deafness, integrated health and living, and legal system. The division helped establish the Foundation for Rehabilitation Psychology, a nonprofit organization supporting research and education in rehabilitation psychology as a means to improve the lives of persons with disabilities. During the late 1970s and 1980s, growth in the area of neurorehabilitation led to a marked increase in the number of rehabilitation psychologists treating persons with brain injury and other neurological disorders. As a result, there is a large overlap of rehabilitation psychology and neuropsychology in this area, and many psychologists self-identify with both specialties or, as Larson and Sachs (2000) note, report that they work in the hybrid of "neuropsychological rehabilitation." Nearly half (49% in 2010) of the Division 22 members are also members of Division 40 (Division of Clinical Neuropsychology), and the two divisions often cosponsor activities at the APA Annual Convention.

The *Division 22 Newsletter* has published interviews with several leaders in the field (Brownsberger, 2004; Homaifar, 2007; Lopez, 2005) that provide historical perspectives about the development of the division, supplemented by the personal thoughts and recollections of significant players in its establishment and growth.

The evolution of the field did not stop with the establishment of an APA division. The growth of the field and the division, as well as the increasing opportunities for rehabilitation psychologists in the job market, again raised the question, "Who is a rehabilitation psychologist?" Organizations such as the Commission for Accreditation of Rehabilitation Facilities (CARF) mandated inclusion of psychologists on inpatient rehabilitation teams. These developments, combined with increased entry into the field of psychologists from a variety of backgrounds (e.g., clinical, counseling, educational, health, neuropsychology), provided an impetus for further attempts to answer the above question.

This led to calls for more specialized education and training (Elliott and Gramling, 1990), including core training; however, there remained a general view that rehabilitation psychology did not require distinct and separate specialty training (e.g., apart from clinical or counseling psychology) at the predoctoral level. Internship and postdoctoral training remained the route for specializing in rehabilitation psychology. Shontz and Wright (1980) laid out some areas of core study for potential rehabilitation psychology programs. However, Cox, Hess, Hibbard, Layman, and Stewart (2010) noted that there is movement toward an emphasis on postdoctoral training becoming the norm, reporting only 8 specialized doctoral programs, over 70 internship sites, and 28 postdoctoral residency (fellowship) programs.

Establishment of Specialty Certification

As Larson and Sachs (2000) point out, credentialing in a professional specialty area is often viewed as a hallmark of that area's maturation. In the early 1990s, led by the Division of Rehabilitation Psychology, the field began to explore whether a desire and/or need existed to more clearly delineate rehabilitation psychology as a specialty area and *rehabilitation psychologists* as specialists. A specialty credentialing committee was established to review this area and make recommendations. A consensus quickly developed that the need and interest existed.

That committee met multiple times each year over a period of several years to discuss and define fundamental rehabilitation psychology principles and practices. Ultimately the committee metamorphosed in 1995 into the American Board of Rehabilitation Psychology (ABRP), incorporated in the state of Missouri. The establishment of specialty board certification in rehabilitation psychology was led by Richard Cox, and the others involved were Bernard Brucker, Bruce Caplan, David Cox, Harry Parker, Anthony Ricci, Daniel Rohe, Mitchell Rosenthal, James Whelan, and Mary Willmuth. Preparing to seek affiliation with the American

Board of Professional Psychology (ABPP), the group identified aspects of the specialty area that were unique to the field and those shared with other areas of psychology, as well as elements that were required for adequate education, training, and experience. The process of translating these areas into specific competencies as defined by the broader psychological arena (e.g., APA, 2006) is dynamic and ongoing (Cox et al., 2010; Hibbard and Cox, 2010).

In 1995, Division 22 voted to support, in spirit as well as through provision of some funding, the ABRP application to the ABPP for affiliation as a specialty area. The first examinations of rehabilitation psychologists by the ABRP were held in 1996 under the "monitoring phase" of ABPP affiliation; that group was granted ABPP board certification upon the ABRP becoming a fully affiliated member board of the ABPP in 1997. In 2008, Division 22 awarded the Lifetime Practice Excellence Award to the founding members of the ABRP in honor of their efforts and achievements. To date, roughly 150 psychologists have become board certified in rehabilitation psychology. In the most recent development, members of the ABRP have begun to establish the Academy of Rehabilitation Psychology, whose fundamental purposes are education and advocacy.

The founding group of the ABRP, as well as those who became board members in later years, envisioned more than simply a board certification process for psychologists engaged in rehabilitation psychology. They took to heart a mission to continue to expand the field, educate its practitioners, and help establish a firmer foundation for those to come. Toward that end, they sought the establishment of an annual conference as well as a charitable foundation for the purpose of advancing rehabilitation psychology. Both of these, in cooperation with Division 22, have come to fruition.

Rehabilitation Psychology: The Division 22/American Board of Rehabilitation Psychology Joint Conference

The ABRP and Division 22 joined forces in 1999 to establish a conference specifically oriented toward education and opportunities for collegial interaction among rehabilitation psychologists. The annual meeting, known simply as Rehabilitation Psychology XXXX (with XXXX denoting the year of the conference), has shown solid growth, providing updates on current research and clinical care in rehabilitation psychology. Historically occurring in March or April, yet more recently set in the last week of February, and attracting 200 to 250 participants, the conference is large enough to be financially feasible yet small enough to permit considerable interaction among those in attendance. Several invited lectures in honor of significant leaders in rehabilitation psychology have been established: the Beatrice Wright and Tamara Dembo Lecture in Rehabilitation Psychology, the Leonard Diller Lecture, and the Rosenthal Memorial Lecture.

An integral part of the conference format has been the establishment of a multitrack ABRP preparation workshop with an introductory portion dealing with the early stages of learning about the process of ABRP certification, and an advanced segment addressing issues germane to those already in the process of preparing practice samples and/or readying for the oral examination. Furthermore, the conference always provides time for those interested in the ABRP to speak with potential mentors for guidance about the ABRP application and evaluation process.

Where the Field Is Headed

Rehabilitation psychology has the double-edged distinction of growing, at least in part, as a result of world conflict and injury. The present day is no different in that regard; the numerous returning veterans with acquired (sometimes multiple) disabilities have yet again given reason to refocus and redouble efforts in rehabilitation psychology (Cox et al., 2010). Injuries sustained by troops serving in Iraq and Afghanistan (Operation Iraqi Freedom and Operation Enduring Freedom) have driven home to the U.S. government and Department of Veterans Affairs the tremendous need for psychological services for veterans and their families. Brenner, Vanderploeg, and Terrio (2009) provided one of the several articles that addressed these and related issues in the journal *Rehabilitation Psychology*. Although this realm of clinical care is highlighted due to current circumstances, it goes without saying that injuries, chronic illness, and disability continue in other areas of society as well. As the population of the United States (and other countries) is aging, there is an increasing demand for services from psychologists well trained in treating illnesses and conditions that afflict the elderly, as well as in assisting with familial and community adaptation, accommodation, and integration (Lichtenberg & Schneider, 2010).

Psychologists in rehabilitation have been integrally involved in developing the International Classification of Functioning, Disability and Health (ICF; World Health Organization, 2001). Further, as has been pointed out elsewhere (e.g., Frank, Gluck, and Buckelew, 1990; Lollar, 2008), rehabilitation psychologists are well suited to assist in research and advocacy in the establishment of public health policy. To paraphrase the early rehabilitation psychology pioneers, as a relatively young psychological specialty, rehabilitation psychology has gained much from other areas of psychology and has much to give to the profession.

Recently, a conference of those involved in the education and training of rehabilitation psychologists aimed to establish more formal and specific direction regarding the pathway to expertise in the field, inclusive of attaining board certification through the ABPP in rehabilitation psychology.

The Baltimore Conference on Rehabilitation Psychology Postdoctoral Training was held in Baltimore, Maryland, in April 2011. The participants were 46 health care professionals from 18 states, including 12 universities, 7 hospitals, 7 Department of Defense and Veterans Administration medical centers and offices, and the American Psychological Association.

These participants represented the American Psychological Association, Division of Rehabilitation Psychology officers, sections, students, early career members, committees, and special interest groups, as well as the American Board of Rehabilitation Psychology, the Academy of Rehabilitation Psychology, the Foundation for Rehabilitation Psychology, the American Psychological Association Education Directorate, and medical education.

The 3-day conference began to develop consensus guidelines on how postdoctoral training programs in rehabilitation psychology should be conducted and the competencies that should be developed, and created the structure for a national organization of postdoctoral training programs in rehabilitation psychology. As of this writing, two publications have arisen from this conference (Stiers, Barisa, et al., in press; Stiers, Hanson, et al., 2012). The guidelines will be published in the near future. Furthermore, the Council of Rehabilitation Psychology Postdoctoral Training Programs held an initial meeting at the Rehabilitation Psychology Conference in February of 2012.

CONCLUSION

Scherer, et al. (2010, p. 1444) summed up rehabilitation psychology as follows:

> Rehabilitation psychologists are uniquely trained and specialized to engage in a broad range of activities that include clinical practice, consultation, program development, service provision, research, teaching and education, training, administration, development of

public policy, and advocacy related to persons with disability and chronic health conditions.

The developments discussed in this chapter offer considerable promise for the further development and professionalization of rehabilitation psychology. Increases in employment opportunities, clinical research, and establishment of accepted guidelines for education and training characterize the likely future of this multifaceted psychological specialty.

PART II

Foundational Competencies

TWO

Ethical and Legal Issues

Constituting substantially—but not entirely—overlapping domains, ethics and legal issues are major concerns of professional psychology practice. What seems ethical may not always be consistent with the law, and what one can do legally may strike the practitioner as at least vaguely unethical. Rehabilitation psychologists are not exempt from responsibility for being familiar with professional ethics codes and the laws of the venues in which they practice. As with other psychological specialties, although there is a substantial shared knowledge base, the nuances and implications for rehabilitation psychologists of ethical strictures and legal statutes are somewhat idiosyncratic. For example, no other specialty must be as conversant with federal legislation that has focused on the needs of persons with a disability. Although one need not be a psychologist or even involved in health care to know that the acronym ADA stands for the Americans With Disabilities Act, the rehabilitation psychologist must be aware of recent decisions that affect how the law is interpreted and applied in specific instances so as to advise and counsel his or her patients effectively. In the realm of ethics, rehabilitation has historically been a team enterprise (Butt & Caplan, 2010)—with an emphasis on sharing of information—which has meant that psychologists practicing in such settings must constantly deal with ethical conundrums concerning such topics as patient confidentiality and patients' thoughts of self-harm.

This chapter focuses on selected areas of ethics and law with which a rehabilitation psychologist should be conversant to some degree. The chapter contains three major sections: (a) an overview of the American Psychological Association (APA) "Ethical Principles of Psychologists and

Code of Conduct," (b) an overview of some of the major laws of which rehabilitation psychologists should be aware, and (c) a brief discussion of some clinical issues that may give rise to ethical and/or legal concerns.

This chapter is *not* intended to be a tutorial on law and ethics, nor comprehensive in nature. Rather, readers should gain from this text a basic familiarity with the topics and then actively contemplate what gaps exist in their own knowledge base, given the specifics of their practice and populations served. For example, the relevance of the ADA may differ as a function of settings (e.g., inpatient care vs. outpatient vocational counseling regarding occupational accommodations for a person with a disability). The nuances of the interaction of law, ethics, and practice of rehabilitation psychology vary widely across settings, populations, and locales. It is the ethical responsibility of the individual rehabilitation psychologist to maintain adequate knowledge of how these may apply in one's practice.

Ethical Principles of Psychologists and Code of Conduct of the American Psychological Association

All competent psychologists are aware of the "Ethical Principles of Psychologists and Code of Conduct" of the APA (2002). Often referred to as the "APA Ethics Code," this document is referenced in the bylaws, legislative language, and/or rules and regulations of many, if not most, organizations, licensing agencies, and other agencies involved in professional psychology. For most psychologists, awareness of and adherence to the APA Ethics Code are routine parts of practice. Indeed, a member of the APA, a psychologist who is board certified through the American Board of Professional Psychology (ABPP), and a psychologist licensed in a jurisdiction that relies on the APA Ethics Code each have independent obligations to their respective organizations or certifying/licensing boards to know and abide by the APA Ethics Code.

The APA Ethics Code is constructed around 5 basic "General Principles" and 10 "Ethical Standards" (there are subsections of the standards). The General Principles are *aspirational* in nature; they are values to be integrated into behavior and practice. They are not obligations and are not enforceable; in other words, the General Principles are not applied to actual situations to determine whether one acted ethically in a given situation, nor are they to be used in sanctioning psychologists. The Ethical Standards, on the other hand, are enforceable. It is the application of the Ethical Standards that results in decision making about activities that might violate the APA Ethics Code. The 5 General Principles (Beneficence and Nonmaleficence,

Fidelity and Responsibility, Integrity, Justice, and Respect for People's Rights and Dignity) and 10 Ethical Standards (Resolving Ethical Issues, Competence, Human Relations, Privacy and Confidentiality, Advertising and Other Public Statements, Record Keeping and Fees, Education and Training, Research and Publication, Assessment, and Therapy) are briefly described in the following sections; rehabilitation psychologists are expected to be familiar with all of these.

THE GENERAL PRINCIPLES

Principle A: Beneficence and Nonmaleficence

One might reasonably describe this principle as "work to benefit others and, above all, do no harm." Psychologists attempt to maximize their benefit to others and minimize harm through awareness of the influence that they have on other people, research animals, organizations, and situations. They guard against detriment to others that may arise from their direct interactions or influence. Psychologists attempt to resolve conflicts responsibly and with minimal negative impact. They strive to be aware of the effects that their own health—physical and mental—may have on others. In their work with persons with disabilities—individuals who may be marginalized by others and/or society at large—rehabilitation psychologists often actively engage in advocacy for the benefit of those whom they serve.

Principle B: Fidelity and Responsibility

Psychologists are expected to be responsible and trustworthy. They attempt to make clear their role(s) and limitations in all situations. They consult with others cooperatively and promote ethical behavior among their colleagues. When questions or concerns about professional matters arise, psychologists consult with other professionals to ascertain how to proceed. A portion of a psychologist's professional time is spent providing services explicitly for the good of others, with little or no remuneration, financial or otherwise. Rehabilitation psychologists are often involved in volunteer work with organizations that advocate for, or provide services to, persons with disabilities

Principle C: Integrity

Rehabilitation psychologists strive to provide honest, accurate, and scientifically sound input to others. They do not intentionally misrepresent facts, lie, cheat, steal, or engage in fraud. The trust that is a core of the relationship that they have with others is a foundation upon which others can rely. Although rehabilitation psychologists may find themselves in situations where they can influence an outcome (e.g., as might arise in legal proceedings that could result in a financial settlement for a client with recent-onset disability), the core value of integrity mandates that such influence is based on honest representation of facts, and opinions are provided based on sound science and professionalism.

Principle D: Justice

Equality and fairness to all persons are notions endorsed by rehabilitation psychologists. This includes using judgment to ensure that the effects of their psychological input and personal biases do not unduly influence others and outcomes. Rehabilitation psychologists are aware of the limitations of their competence, and therefore consult with, or refer to, others when faced with unfamiliar clinical situations.

Principle E: Respect for People's Rights and Dignity

Rehabilitation psychologists maintain confidentiality and respect the rights of others. They are particularly sensitive to the limitations of those they serve, as well as negative societal stereotypes about persons with disabilities, and apply additional safeguards to ensure that the rights of persons with disabilities are protected. They are attuned to differences that arise based on age, culture, sexual orientation, and other such variables; furthermore, they attempt to eliminate or minimize the effects that their own biases may have on others.

The General Principles are clearly provided to guide psychologists in a fashion that will maximize the benefits to others and society at large. At times, reasonable people may disagree about the extent to which the principles have been properly applied. Competency in rehabilitation psychology involves recognizing this, accepting the ambiguity, and being willing to engage in reasonable and respectful discourse with others about alternative points of view.

THE ETHICAL STANDARDS

The 10 overarching Ethical Standards are briefly described in the following paragraphs. The descriptions largely include information from each of the various subcategories, but rehabilitation psychologists should refer directly to the APA Ethics Code for details of the Ethical Standards. It is advisable to keep a copy readily accessible for reference as needed. As rehabilitation psychologists strive to uphold the General Principles, it is imperative that they maintain familiarity with the details of the Ethical

Standards, including revisions that occur over time. Of note: Some important amendments have been recently made, and these are specifically referenced in the paragraph prefaced "Updated."

Standard 1: Resolving Ethical Issues

When aware of misuse or misrepresentation of their work, psychologists seek to correct the situation. They express a commitment to the APA Ethics Code and work to find appropriate resolution. Psychologists work with others informally to resolve conflicts and violations whenever possible. It is expected that informal steps to resolve concerns are taken *prior to* formal reporting of a violation. Direct consultation with the individual psychologist with whom one has a concern is an expected initial step. When informal resolution is not achieved, and when the violation is believed to have caused harm or is likely to do so, formal reporting is made to state or national committees, licensing agencies, and/or certifying agencies. Psychologists cooperate with ethics committees in investigations and proceedings. They do not file unfounded complaints. They do not discriminate against others against whom a complaint has been filed; they base their actions on the outcome of appropriate proceedings and recognize the difference between a filed complaint and a finding of violation.

Updated: The 2002 Ethics Code Standard 1.02 Conflicts Between Ethics and Law, Regulations, or Other Governing Legal Authority and Standard 1.03 Conflicts Between Ethics and Organizational Demands have recently been amended. Prior language in the Ethics Code provided for adherence to governing laws or regulations and included language that might be perceived as more ambiguous (e.g., "to the extent feasible") than the amended Ethics Code. The language has been recently changed to reflect that psychologists are to attempt to find resolutions that preserve basic principles of human rights and that prohibit use of the standard in "justifying or defending" human rights violations (APA, 2010a).

Standard 2: Competence

Psychologists work within their area(s) of competence, continuously engage in activities that help to maintain competence, and base their work on scientific and professional knowledge of psychology. The may, in emergency situations, engage in activities that are beyond their training when others who are suitably trained are unavailable; however, they cease provision of these services as soon as possible. In rural areas or small towns, which tend to be far removed from rehabilitation facilities, a general clinical psychologist, although lacking specific training in rehabilitation psychology, may be called upon to treat individuals with disabilities. In such cases, the psychologist can seek remote supervision and digest relevant contemporary literature.

When working with and/or supervising others, it is incumbent on the psychologist to establish that those others also are working within their level of competence. Psychologists do not delegate to others work for which those others may not be competent. They are vigilant about the possible effects of multiple relationships, as well as the possibility that their personal problems may compromise competent provision of services.

Because training programs in rehabilitation psychology are still few in number, many clinicians come to work in rehabilitation settings with little formal training or experience with conditions commonly encountered there such as spinal cord injury, stroke, or brain injury. From their first day on the job, newcomers to the specialty should endeavor to bolster their knowledge through targeted readings, consultation with more experienced colleagues, and continuing education.

Standard 3: Human Relations

Psychologists do not engage in unfair discrimination based on age, gender, culture, or other individual difference factors. Sexual and other forms of harassment or behavior that may be demeaning to others are not knowingly practiced by psychologists. The adage "do no harm" applies to all with whom the psychologist engages and extends to individuals, animals, research participants, and organizations alike. The existence of multiple relationships is recognized by psychologists and is considered thoughtfully. There may be times when it is difficult or impossible to avoid multiple relationships. For example, rehabilitation psychologists frequently provide services to spouses, children, or other significant individuals in the patient's social network. This typically occurs after involvement with the patient on an individual basis. When services are expanded in this way, psychologists clarify the boundaries of their role and attempt to minimize adverse effect on others. Conflicts of interest, financial or otherwise, are avoided. Psychologists clarify with others *at the onset of services* who the client is and the nature of the psychologist's relationships with others. Exploitation of others is prohibited, and it is expected that psychologists cooperate with other professionals. Services and activities are provided after obtaining the informed consent of those involved. This includes describing the nature of services, limitations of the services, limitations of confidentiality, and other factors. Psychologists attempt to minimize the effects that may arise should illness or other issues interrupt services.

Standard 4: Privacy and Confidentiality

It is a primary obligation of psychologists to maintain confidentiality, discuss the limits of confidentiality, and maintain records in a fashion that protects confidentiality. Efforts are made to minimize provision of private information in reports and otherwise, unless that information is necessary. Legal and other situations may arise in which it is acceptable to disclose some confidential information; this can be permissible, but it is done in a fashion that minimizes disclosure to the level required for the circumstance. Reasonable steps are made to prevent disclosing personally identifiable information in situations such as reporting of case information in research, writing, and teaching. Due to the importance of participation in a rehabilitation treatment team approach (Butt & Caplan, 2010), rehabilitation psychologists frequently face circumstances in which privacy and confidentiality issues arise. As such, they engage in ongoing review of what is and is not germane to be disclosed in any given situation, and they consult with others when uncertain.

Standard 5: Advertising and Other Public Statements

Psychologists avoid the use of false, misleading, and/or deceptive advertising or public statements; they maintain responsibility for statements made by others they engage to represent them. Psychologists who are responsible for brochures or announcements strive to ensure accuracy in representation of programs and other information in the materials. Statements made in the media by psychologists are to be based on professional experience and training, grounded in the psychological literature and consistent with the Ethics Code. Psychologists do not solicit testimonials from others who may be vulnerable to undue influence.

Although many, if not most, rehabilitation psychologists have or will acquire some skill in health psychology concepts and practices and in neuropsychological assessment, one needs to be cognizant of the difference between having some skills in an area and having the level of competency that specialists in that area deem necessary to hold oneself out to the public as a "heath psychologist" or "clinical neuropsychologist."

Standard 6: Record Keeping and Fees

Professional and scientific work conducted by a psychologist is recorded in compliance with the Ethics Code and requirements of state and/or other appropriate regulating authorities. Records are kept securely and confidentially and are released when requisite consent is obtained. Fees and payment arrangements are discussed clearly and completely as early as possible in the professional relationship and are not misrepresented. Attempts to collect fees due using collection agencies or other legal means are discussed with the person who owes the fees, and the person is provided an opportunity to make payment prior to initiation of such activity. Bartering, if conducted, is generally frowned upon and must be considered carefully based on potential clinical contraindications, consideration of multiple relationships, and the possibility of exploitation. Reports made to payers and funding sources are accurate. Psychologists neither pay fees to nor receive fees from other professionals for providing referrals.

As many individuals become rehabilitation patients through the mechanism of automobile accidents or other traumatic events, it is not uncommon for litigation to occur several years after the fact. This mandates adequate maintenance of records for the period of time required by the jurisdiction in which the psychologist practices. In addition, one must be aware of the possibility of being called to testify at a much later date, should the matter be taken to arbitration, mediation, or trial.

Standard 7: Education and Training

Psychologists prepare workshops and educational and training programs to meet the goals set forth in the program. Descriptions of educational and training materials are maintained so as to be current and accurate, including the requirements necessary for program completion. Teaching, use of student personal information, requirements for mandatory therapy, and student/supervisee performance evaluation are areas that require careful consideration of the Ethics Code. The psychologist involved in these activities must maintain accuracy of materials, consider the real need for personal information, and determine suitable personnel to provide therapy for students or supervisees. Psychologists do not provide therapy services to those whose performance they are to evaluate. Psychologists do not engage in sexual relations with students or supervisees for whom they provide performance evaluations.

Standard 8: Research and Publication

When conducting research and publication activities, required institutional approval and informed consent of individual(s) involved are obtained. The psychologist researcher gives thorough consideration to the implications of his or her relationships with potential participants in order to protect those individuals from negative consequences should they not participate or withdraw from the project. Participants in research are provided an opportunity to obtain information about the research, and results are reported accurately; should errors later be discovered, psychologists attempt to report corrections. Publication credits are made in accordance with actual work done, and psychologists do not engage in plagiarism or duplication (as original data) of data without proper citation of the original work. When conducting review of materials for publications, presentations, or grants, psychologists respect the rights of those who submitted such materials.

Rehabilitation psychologists involved in research often must seek informed consent from individuals whose cognitive functioning is compromised. This does not release the psychologist from the obligation (as a matter of common courtesy, if nothing else) to attempt to explain the situation in terms that can be grasped by the patient, in addition to thoroughly informing a suitable stand-in and securing consent from that individual.

It is also true that some common treatments in rehabilitation psychology do not yet have a solid empirical basis supporting their efficacy but are being studied for their effects on outcome. This, too, needs to be conveyed to recipients of those interventions so that they understand that they may not benefit directly from their participation.

Standard 9: Assessment

Assessment and evaluation activities are conducted using suitable instruments, with opinions reported that are supported by scientific and professional literature and knowledge. Test selection is made for particular populations with an awareness of the existence of validity and reliability for such populations and of the strengths and limitations inherent in the use of the instruments.

Rehabilitation psychologists, in particular, frequently need to evaluate the interaction of the testing procedure and the individual being tested. Nonstandardized approaches to assessment (which, in many cases, simply involves the common practice of "testing the limits") may be called for in order to obtain information being sought, as is addressed briefly in this text and in the writings of Caplan and Shechter (1995, 2005). In any resulting report, deviations from standard procedures should be justified and explained, and the results interpreted with due caution.

The Ethics Code indicates that psychologists obtain informed consent for testing, explaining the nature and purpose of the process using language that can be understood by an individual who may have limited comprehension; interpreter services are used when absolutely necessary with consideration of the potential pitfalls.

Many assessments in rehabilitation settings involve litigation, disability insurance applications, and other reasons that test results may be requested by third parties. In such circumstances, the psychologist should consider whether information that may be solicited would include sensitive personal information that could be misused or misrepresented. It is also important to consider whether complying with a request for information would result in release of test materials that should be kept secure to maintain test integrity and that might be covered by other laws such as copyright and contract law. Prior to releasing information, therefore, it is important that the psychologist carefully consider the differences between and among test *results*, test *data*, and test *materials*. Hanson and Kerkhoff (2010) discuss this issue in the context of a case vignette, including options of obtaining legal/judicial input, redacting some aspects of the record to protect test integrity, and providing limited viewing of the materials under controlled conditions.

Psychologists should rely on tests that are not obsolete and that are useful for the designated assessment purpose. Automated, computerized, external, or other test scoring or interpretation services are used with due consideration of the supporting (and refuting) evidence and the reliability and validity of such services, and with awareness that the psychologist using such services remains ultimately responsible for the selection, use, and interpretation of the tests or assessment tools administered.

Finally, psychologists maintain responsibility to explain the results of assessment to the individual or that person's designee. Certain situations may preclude that, however, such as employment or forensic evaluations. In these situations, a psychologist is responsible for explaining to the person being evaluated the limited nature of the relationship and inherent restrictions in reporting results to that person, as well as explain to whom such results will be reported.

Standard 10: Therapy

When providing therapy, psychologists obtain informed consent and also clarify at the outset of therapy the identity of the client. When multiple parties are involved (e.g., couples or family therapy), the identified client and relationship that the psychologist has with participants are defined; further clarification, modification of, and/or withdrawal from a role may be necessary if possible roles may conflict (as in divorce proceedings). Psychologists similarly clarify roles and responsibilities of all involved in group therapy. If providing services to persons already engaged in similar services elsewhere, the psychologist discusses this with the client and consults with the other service provider(s) as indicated. Psychologists do not engage in sexual intimacy with clients, their close relatives, or other parties with whom the client has a significant relationship. They do not accept as clients people with whom they have had sexual intimacies, nor do they engage in sexual intimacy with former clients. The APA Ethical Standards provide only for cases of very unusual circumstances as exceptions to this latter item. Careful consideration is given to the client/patient situation in the event that therapy must be interrupted, and steps are taken to provide for effective resolution/transfer of responsibilities and/or termination of therapy. Many, if not most, rehabilitation psychologists work in settings that provide care on a time-limited basis; it is therefore essential that there is adequate planning for, and discussion of, psychological service provision after discharge from that setting.

Legal Issues

Rehabilitation psychologists should have a fundamental awareness of the significant laws that affect their practice and/or the people whom they serve. Although a rehabilitation psychologist is not expected to grasp legal issues as fully as a practicing attorney, the psychologist should understand the laws that are relevant to the services provided. For example, when involved with a patient who wishes to return to work with a new disability, the psychologist should be conversant with laws that may mandate that the employer provide reasonable accommodations to a returning employee. In such situations, the psychologist may consult with the employer prior to, or in conjunction with, the employee's return, thereby serving as both mediator and advocate.

Psychologists can learn more about federal laws related to persons with disabilities by reviewing *A Guide to Disability Rights Laws* by the U.S. Department of Justice (2005). Other legal matters that have to do with state regulations concerning the practice of psychology may be accessed directly from each state jurisdiction through the Association of State and Provincial Psychology Boards (ASPPB) website (http://www.asppb.net). The ASPPB's membership is composed primarily of licensing boards of the states, Canadian provinces, and U.S. territories. Links to the licensing boards as well as relevant jurisdictional laws, categorized by jurisdiction, can be found on the ASPPB website. Psychologists are well advised to utilize this site as a launching point from which to access laws, regulations, and related state licensing board materials.

SOME IMPORTANT FEDERAL LEGISLATION PERTINENT TO REHABILITATION PSYCHOLOGY

Rehabilitation Act of 1973 (Public Law 93–112)

The Rehabilitation Act of 1973 was a major step forward in legislation affecting persons with disabilities. This federal law prohibits discrimination on the basis of disability, provides for affirmative action steps, prohibits denial of benefits or exclusion from programs based on disability, and specifies requirements for accessibility of information through adaptive/assistive technology. The law applies to federal agencies as well as those that contract with the federal government and/or receive federal financial assistance. Funding arising from the Rehabilitation Act is a mainstay of vocational rehabilitation programs nationwide (Fraser & Johnson, 2010). Thus, the impact is extensive, and this piece of legislation set the stage for other related laws in the coming years. The Rehabilitation Act of 1973 essentially established civil rights of individuals with disabilities.

Sections 504 and 508 of the Rehabilitation Act had wide-reaching impact. Section 504 provides for educational opportunities for persons with disabilities. The law applies to children and adults alike and directs that reasonable accommodations be made as needed. Section 508 states that information must be made accessible to persons with disabilities through electronic and other technological means; clearly, it is essential that rehabilitation psychologists who work with persons with visual or hearing impairment be familiar with these mandates. This section not only dictated provision of information by way of existing technologies but also directed that technology be developed.

Many technologies that we now take for granted and see or use on a daily basis developed as a direct result of Section 508 of the Rehabilitation Act. For example, ATM machines now provide information through multiple avenues such as visual, auditory, and Braille. The software that magnifies and/or reads what is on a computer screen, for example, grew out of a recognition of technology developers that there was not only a need for such technology but also a federal mandate. Sections 504 and 508 were factors that fostered involvement of organizations such as International Business Machines (IBM) in developing assistive technology and cognitive rehabilitation technologies (Cox & Mahaffey, 1994).

Individuals With Disabilities Education Act

Originally known as the Education for All Handicapped Children Act (EHA), the law was initially enacted as Public Law 94–142 in 1975 and mandated that free, appropriate education would be provided to eligible children with disabilities, with due consideration of individual educational needs. The law has been amended several times since its enactment; in 1990 the name was changed to the Individuals With Disabilities Education Act (IDEA), and it was most recently revised in 2004. That revision is P.L. 108–446, the Individuals With Disabilities Education Improvement Act of 2004. The U.S. Department of Education maintains a website devoted to information about IDEA (http://idea.ed.gov).

IDEA is a cornerstone of rehabilitation consultation with schools and special education services. Rehabilitation psychologists working in, or in consultation with, schools and/or with children should be familiar with the basics of this law. The regulations that make up IDEA include definitions of disabilities and eligibility for services, information pertaining to the requirements for evaluations of children, and guidance for Individual Education Plans (IEPs) and Individual Family Service Plans (IFSPs), as well provisions for funding of early intervention services (Flanagan & Miller, 2010).

Related to educational services, but independent of IDEA, rehabilitation psychologists working with individuals in school settings should also be aware of the Family Education Rights and Privacy Act (FERPA) of 1974 that grants rights for review of educational records to individuals age 18 or older as well as to parents of children younger than 18.

Americans With Disabilities Act

Passed in 1990 as Public Law 101–336, the Americans With Disabilities Act (ADA) was an outgrowth of the Rehabilitation Act of 1973. The law provides for equal opportunity and nondiscrimination for individuals with disabilities in employment, occupational settings, public areas such as public buildings and public transportation, and governmental agencies (Bruyère & O'Keefe, 1994). Current information can be accessed through the website (http://www.ada.gov). The ADA is probably the most significant law regarding civil rights for persons with disabilities, promoting "…normalization, empowerment and maximal community integration of individuals with disabilities" (Hibbard & Cox, 2010, pp. 468–469).

Due to its wide-reaching effects and implications, the ADA is frequently found as an issue on court dockets. The law is written fairly broadly to cover the rights of persons with disabilities, attempting to remove barriers that might prevent them from engaging in "major life activities." The law also includes language that covers individuals who have a physical or mental disability, have records of having had such a disability, or are regarded as having such. Clearly, then, this law can conceivably apply to many individuals. As such, there have been numerous cases with importance for rehabilitation psychology. Some such cases have concluded that factors including treatment (e.g., anticonvulsant medication) can mitigate what might otherwise be a disabling condition, while implying that noncompliance with treatment (which thereby perpetuates the condition) can be grounds for denying an individual certain benefits (http://library.findlaw.com/1999/Jun/1/128673.html). It is well beyond the scope of this chapter to address these issues in detail, and the rehabilitation psychologist may not confront them on a day-to-day basis. However, rehabilitation psychologists should be aware that there are frequent and ongoing challenges to the ADA in the form of cases that refine and redefine the law.

Health Information Portability and Accountability Act

The Health Information Portability and Accountability Act (HIPAA) of 1996 affects rehabilitation psychologists in a variety of ways. The law was enacted to protect privacy of patient information as well as to facilitate secure transfer of information to improve the overall health system in the United States. A portion of the law addresses *privacy* and another addresses *security* (U.S. Department of Health & Human Services, 2003). The former is a set of standards regarding protection of specific health information, while the latter sets forth standards for health information that is held in electronic form. Clearly, because rehabilitation psychologists work with health information and often have such information in electronic form, *both* aspects of HIPAA apply.

The relation between HIPAA and the APA Ethics Code has been addressed by Behnke (2005) and by Hanson and Kerkhoff (2010). They point out that the requirement to permit access to health information and the ethical obligations of psychologists may occasionally be at odds with one another. For example, providing access to health information may compete with an ethical obligation to protect test security.

Rehabilitation psychologists need to be aware that HIPAA affects their practice in some rather simple ways, but also in ways that may exceed their expertise. For example, it is relatively easy for a rehabilitation psychologist to use programs and information readily available from sources such as the APA and HIPAA-compliant forms for use in the office; however, complying with the HIPAA security rules may require technological savvy that some psychologists do not have. Rehabilitation psychologists are well advised to familiarize themselves with HIPAA through programs such as the APA HIPAA for Psychologists continuing education program (APA, 2010b) and to seek additional consultation as appropriate.

ADDITIONAL EXAMPLES OF ETHICAL AND LEGAL ISSUES

Social Security and Other Disability Insurance

Rehabilitation psychologists are frequently requested to comment on disability for the purposes of Social Security Disability Insurance (SSDI) or other insurers. It is important in such cases that the psychologist be aware of the difference between *disability* as it may be used in the strictly clinical sense and *disability* as used in public/private policy, rule, regulation, and law. In such cases, the term *disability* is a contractually defined term that may vary from policy to policy. Determination of disability in these cases is not a *clinical* decision; rather, it is an *administrative* determination made by using clinical information and applying it to the specific language of the disability insurance contract. This is frequently misunderstood by psychologists and persons applying for disability benefits alike, yet it is a critical distinction. Also, psychologists are typically constrained (due to ethics, experience/training, and/or policy/rule/regulatory/legal language) to commenting on the *psychological* issues relative to a disability determination yet often overstep this in reports provided to the Social Security Administration (SSA) and other carriers. Rehabilitation psychologists should obtain training and education in determination of disability in order to appreciate the variations of this type of administrative decision making versus conventional clinical assessment. An overview of assessment of disability, with particular focus on the context of the SSA rules, is provided by Cox and Goldberg (2010).

Person-First Language

Although use of person-first language may not technically be an ethical obligation or a legal requirement, it is an important issue to many persons with disabilities. Furthermore, because cultural awareness is in the APA Ethics Code, it seems appropriate to address this here. The concept is a rather simple one. "Person-first language" references the person first and then the descriptor. For example, one does not work with "a brain-injured person," but rather with "a person with a brain injury." To some, this may seem a trivial distinction, and others may find the phrasing awkward or contorted, but because language shapes our concepts, using person-first language promotes a more health-oriented humanizing view of persons with disabilities (Caplan, 1995).

Competency/Capacity

Rehabilitation psychologists may find themselves asked to make judgments about competency or capacity. First and foremost, the rehabilitation psychologist should be familiar with state and federal laws related to *competency*, a legal term that is related to, but not the same as, *capacity*, which is a clinical term. The two terms are often used interchangeably, however, and rehabilitation psychologists should understand and educate others about the differences. Reviewing case vignettes such as those in the volume by Bush (2005) should prove of value in this effort. Limitations of test instruments and their relation to everyday activities (i.e., ecological validity) such as driving or managing finances needs to be considered, as do other factors such as response bias (in the circumstances of pending civil or criminal litigation).

Competency/capacity issues can arise in several forms, and rehabilitation psychologists may find themselves involved in cases that vary greatly from one another (Wood & Kubik, 2005). Typical areas in which questions of competence/capacity arise include criminal and/or civil litigation, informed consent, ability to make decisions, ability to care for oneself independently, right to refuse treatment, and evaluations involving safety and judgment such as driving and some occupational areas, among others. It is important for rehabilitation psychologists in acute inpatient settings to understand that they may be working with an individual whose capacity for informed decision making is so compromised as to raise doubts about his or her ability to provide informed consent.

Additional Areas of Consideration

The array of situations in which rehabilitation psychologists may find themselves faced with ethical and/or legal decisions is seemingly unlimited. These include end-of-life care, ability to sign legal documents, preparation of wills, parenting skills, ability to drive, decision making regarding such topics as "do not resuscitate," guardianship versus self-determination, assessment of malingering/symptom exaggeration/response bias, the role of faith and religion in a patient's decision making, and so forth. Dilemmas are not always of critical clinical importance, yet they may exist nonetheless, and thoughtfulness, consultation, and well-reasoned decisions are essential. Having an established rationale for one's professional decision making, based on careful consideration of ethical and legal issues, is therefore quite important. Hanson and Kerkhoff (2010) offer an overview of several models of ethical decision making, and it is advised that rehabilitation psychologists review decision-making models in evaluating their own response to ethical and/or legal issues.

THREE

Individual and Cultural Diversity

American society is no longer viewed as a "melting pot" but rather as a "tossed salad." The concept of individuals and groups merging their behavioral patterns and beliefs into one shared set of "American" cultural norms has yielded to an appreciation of the numerous differences that characterize our society. This diversity encompasses factors such as ethnicity, race, age, gender, sexual orientation, religion, political views, geography, and other variables that combine and interact with other (perhaps less readily identifiable) individual and/or familial differences. Of greatest relevance to the present chapter, "disability" has come to be viewed as another "diversity" characteristic (Olkin, 2002). As educational programs in African-American studies and women's or gender studies emerged some years ago, recent times have witnessed the emergence of programs in disability studies.

Diversity extends across groups as well as individuals, and an understanding of an individual cannot be based on group descriptors any more than a group could be adequately described by the characteristics of one member. Although this may seem quite obvious, the need for psychologists to consider diversity factors has not always been so clear. The evolution of the field has led to an explicit recognition of the pitfalls of insufficient awareness of diversity and a greater focus on training for, and competency in, psychological work with people of diverse backgrounds.

Rehabilitation psychology has historically been grounded in a biopsychosocial approach that acknowledges the fundamental importance of individual–environment interaction. This focus derives largely from the work of Beatrice Wright and her colleagues, who described the importance of psychological and social interaction in rehabilitation efforts

(Dembo, Leviton, & Wright, 1956; Wright, 1960). A passage from Wright's early writing about rehabilitation psychology, although specifically about disability, could easily apply to the various parameters of diversity:

> With respect to the attitudes of the professional person, it was acknowledged that students of psychology, like anyone else, carry emotional attitudes toward disability, some of which—aversion, fear, or pity, for instance—interfere with sound relations to clients. It was also acknowledged that myths and fancies regarding the psychological significance of disability are legion, and that the psychologist, unless made aware of these misconceptions, would fall prey to them (Wright, 1959, p.60).

Psychological education and training have incorporated major efforts to ensure consideration of diversity, to foster awareness and competency, and to decrease untoward biases (American Psychological Association [APA], 2003; Davis-Russell, Forbes, Bascuas, & Duran, 1991). La Roche and Christopher (2010) point out that the process of integrating cultural competency into psychology as a field, as well as within an individual practitioner's frame of reference, is an evolutionary one. This evolution involves moving from defining the *content* of relevant issues to determining *processes* that may help bridge the gap between practitioner and client when diversity exists.

Integrating diversity competency into the practice of rehabilitation psychology requires recognition of the many areas of potential difference between the practitioner and client such as those mentioned earlier. However, a list of factors that might differ between groups and/or individuals could be seemingly endless, and some differences may not have any actual significance. An awareness of the possibility (if not probability) of cultural differences between individuals and/or groups is at least as important for the rehabilitation psychologist as is the ability to list the differences.

Much literature on diversity, therefore, addresses *cultural* competency in a way that attempts to encompass both interpersonal and intergroup differences. This includes defining culture as the shared constructs, meanings, and beliefs that arise from the array of communications, symbols, and knowledge passed along from generation to generation (Ortiz & Dynda, 2010). La Roche and Christopher (2010) utilize a similar definition (that of Geertz, 1973) that adequately addresses issues of diversity of racial, ethnic, and disability status, among others.

Lakes, Lopez, and Garro (2006) address cultural competence through a case example, illustrating how learning about another's culture in the context of a larger social system, as well as that individual's life story, can enhance the clinician's ability to understand and intervene effectively. The article reviews the case of a child with a developmental disability who has been sexually abused. Although not specifically identified as a *rehabilitation* psychology case, it includes a number of diversity issues that a rehabilitation psychologist may encounter and offers a means of appreciating some of the various models for understanding cultural competence. An article by Kerkhoff and Hanson (2007) centers around the case of a Latino adolescent with a traumatic brain injury during whose rehabilitation stay cultural factors were not adequately taken into account. The authors offer suggestions for better management of cultural differences in light of the APA multicultural and ethical guidelines. These case vignettes bear some resemblance to those that rehabilitation psychologists might encounter in pursuing board certification in rehabilitation psychology through the American Board of Rehabilitation Psychology (ABRP).

It is important not only that psychologists have multicultural knowledge but also that they be aware of ways in which their own perspective may shape their perceptions of others and take steps to minimize or eliminate any detrimental distorting effects that their own viewpoints may bring to interpersonal interactions. Fields (2010) presents two case vignettes illustrating how Type I and Type II errors (incorrect acceptance/rejection of, in this case, the hypothesis that culture is the contributing variable) can cause psychologists to err when unaware of their own cultural expectations, beliefs, and views. Interaction between client and psychologist can serve to improve the mutual understanding of cultural views and provide effective corrective action at times as each begins to use the narrative more fully to understand the other (La Roche & Christopher, 2010).

Vasquez (2007) reviewed cultural influences on effectiveness of psychotherapy, issues regarding establishment of and threats to therapeutic alliance, and biases that a psychologist may have. She also reported briefly on unintentional bias and underlying neuroscience findings (Eberhardt, 2005) that suggest that neural pathways involved in negative biases might be subject to change and that future research may reveal that neuroanatomical group differences are associated with social and/or cultural factors.

DIVERSITY, AMERICAN PSYCHOLOGICAL ASSOCIATION ETHICS CODE, AND AMERICAN PSYCHOLOGICAL ASSOCIATION MULTICULTURAL GUIDELINES

The APA Multicultural Guidelines use "diversity" as a rather broad term including social identities, sexual orientation, age, gender, and more (APA, 2003, p. 380). For the purposes of this chapter, "diversity" is used loosely to refer to the larger scope of cultural, racial, ethnic, and multicultural diversity factors. The issue of diversity is formally addressed within ethical principles and standards for psychologists as well as guidelines put forth by the APA. Given that psychologists are often held to these by their state and/or national organizations as well as the licensing board in their jurisdictions, it is important that they be aware of the specifics. Therefore, they are addressed directly herein.

The American Psychological Association Ethics Code and Diversity Issues

In the "Ethical Principles of Psychologists and Code of Conduct" (APA, 2002), Principle E: Respect for People's Rights and Dignity, addresses the basic respect that psychologists should demonstrate for the dignity and worth of all people, including the rights of individuals. The principle emphasizes the ethical importance of cultural awareness, respect for differences/diversity, and the aspiration that psychologists try to minimize or eliminate the effects on their work of their own biases. Several differences are specified: age, gender, gender identity, race, ethnicity, culture, national origin, religion, sexual orientation, disability, language, and socioeconomic status. However, it is also clear that this is not necessarily intended to be an exhaustive list.

Rehabilitation psychologists need to familiarize themselves thoroughly with the APA Ethics Code. Although the verbatim text of the Ethics Code is not given here, a number of the sections are described *as examples* of those of which one should be aware and with which one should be in compliance. The Standards (in contrast to the Principles) of the APA Ethics Code are enforceable (i.e., one can be sanctioned for not complying with the Standards).

Some areas in which competence with respect to diversity is noted in the APA Ethics Code include:

> Ethical Standard 2: Competence
> *Section 2.01(b): Boundaries of Competence*

This section references the need for psychologists to have appropriate training, experience, consultation, and/or supervision when providing services that can require an understanding of diversity issues. For example, a psychologist working with a patient with a recent spinal cord injury should be familiar with the functional implications (including those for sexual expression) of various levels of spine injury, types of common pain complaints, and possibility of coexisting head trauma.

> Ethical Standard 3: Human Relations
> *Section 3.01: Unfair Discrimination*

This section indicates that psychologists do not, in their work-related activities, engage in unfair discrimination based on issues of diversity such as age, gender, race, and so forth.

> *Section 3.03: Other Harassment*

Psychologists do not knowingly engage in behavior that is harassing based on issues of diversity such as age, gender, race, and so forth.

> *Ethical Standard 3.10: Informed Consent*
> *Sections 3.10 (a), (b)*

Informed consent must be obtained using language and whatever means of communication might be necessary to ensure (to the extent possible) that it can be understood by the participant. When an individual is legally incapable of providing informed consent (e.g., because of brain injury–related cognitive impairment or lack of facility in the language of the dominant culture), the psychologist endeavors to obtain it from a person legally authorized to provide consent.

The standard regarding informed consent also applies in relatively similar fashion to some other standards including, but not necessarily limited to, Ethical Standard 9: Assessment and Ethical Standard 10: Therapy.

The American Psychological Association Multicultural Guidelines

The APA has also established Guidelines on Multicultural Education, Training, Research, Practice and Organizational Change for Psychologists, specifically regarding issues of diversity (APA, 2003). (These guidelines are hereinafter referred to as the APA Multicultural Guidelines.) They encourage psychologists to (a) recognize that their own beliefs and attitudes can affect (perhaps detrimentally) their interactions with others, (b) recognize the importance of multicultural sensitivity/responsiveness, and (c) endeavor to incorporate cultural sensitivity/responsiveness into the work that they do in education, research, practice, and organizational processes. The APA Multicultural Guidelines provide a framework for understanding diversity in the various arenas in which psychologists work in addition to offering some review of research, definitions, and examples relevant to the practice of psychology. Defined within the APA Multicultural Guidelines are the terms *culture, race, ethnicity, multiculturalism and diversity, and culture centered.*

The APA Multicultural Guidelines (p. 380) cite Pedersen (1997, p. 256): "If culture is part of the environment, and all behavior is shaped by culture, then culture-centered counseling is responsive to all culturally learned patterns." This is highly reminiscent of the long-standing tradition of rehabilitation psychology's sensitivity to the interaction between an individual with an impairment or a disability and the environment. Wright (1959, pp. 8–9), referencing discussions among herself and colleagues at a seminal institute on rehabilitation psychology, noted the importance of considering the individual in the great context of one's culture:

> It was pointed out that though rehabilitation should take into account or even give special attention to life in the community with its social and physical realities, one should not at the same time exclude other factors of crucial relevance to the rehabilitation outcome. Among those mentioned were conditions influencing adjustment in the hospital situation, the patient's life history, his premorbid personality, his personal attitudes and feelings about his disability.... It was stressed, for instance, that prevention of deeply disturbed emotional reactions in the event of disability inevitably requires attention to attitudes and values that pervade society.

Rehabilitation psychologists should recognize the likelihood that, prior to acquiring their disability, many (if not most) of their patients held attitudes toward persons with disabilities that are prevalent in our society, and many of these tend to be negative and "devaluing" (e.g., Yuker, 1988). At least initially, some persons with disabilities may appear to be "in denial" because of their resistance to self-identifying as "handicapped."

Specifically, the APA Multicultural Guidelines are as follows:

Guideline 1: Psychologists are encouraged to recognize that, as cultural beings, they may hold attitudes and beliefs that can detrimentally influence their perceptions of and interactions with individuals who are ethnically and racially different from themselves.

Guideline 2: Psychologists are encouraged to recognize the importance of multicultural sensitivity/responsiveness to, knowledge of, and understanding about ethnically and racially different individuals.

Guideline 3: As educators, psychologists are encouraged to employ the constructs of multiculturalism and diversity in psychological education.

Guideline 4: Culturally sensitive psychological researchers are encouraged to recognize the importance of conducting culture-centered and ethical psychological research among persons from ethnic, linguistic, and racial minority backgrounds.

Guideline 5: Psychologists are encouraged to apply culturally appropriate skills in clinical and other applied psychological practices.

Guideline 6: Psychologists are encouraged to use organizational change process to support culturally informed organizational (policy) development and practices.

Defining Multicultural Variables

Attempts to define the variety of multicultural variables that might be encountered in practice will inevitably be incomplete. Nonetheless, the literature does contain good resources for some cultures and demographics, with some specifically provided in relation to disability.

Several cultural groups and many of the important values they hold are discussed by Sue and Sue (2007). Understanding the concept of machismo among Latino males or the importance of social deference in some Asian cultures, for example, in contrast to American cultural norms, may be facilitated by such readings. Of particular importance to rehabilitation psychologists are notions about health and disability. For example, Schaller, Parker, and Garcia (1998) pointed out that Mexican immigrant workers do not have a word for disability, and this is also true for many Native American cultures (Mpofu, Beck, & Weinrach, 2004). Some cultures tend to view disability as something that is to be taken care of within the immediate or extended family, may not be aware of rehabilitation services, and may view illness/injury/impairment/disability as a weakness, or perhaps even as a familial curse.

Women and men of the same culture may experience disability differently. Nosek (2010) reports that women with a disability are more likely to live alone, be divorced, and be less well-educated as well as unemployed and impoverished. Individuals who have deeply religious and/or spiritual belief systems may express their disability experience in quite different terms than do atheists or agnostics. In some cases, religious or spiritual beliefs may be viewed as reflecting maladjustment (Albright, Forchheimer, & Tate, 2010) or perhaps even an "antirehabilitation" frame of mind ("It's God's will that I be handicapped."). On the other hand, some with strong religious beliefs will recall that "God helps those who help themselves" and see rehabilitation as a challenge to be met.

Some have pointed out that defining persons with disabilities as a "minority" and "a culture" may well be *statistically* accurate. Artman and Daniels (2010), in addressing cultural competence in provision of psychotherapy to persons with disabilities, point out that the largest single minority in the United States is that of persons with a disability. Mpofu and colleagues (2004) assert that numbers alone do not define minority status, but there are other factors to consider. Social status variables such as access to economic and other benefits, ability to engage in life as one prefers, employment, and other forms of denial of rights and/or discrimination may be readily observed when reviewing what is part and parcel of the culture (desired or not) of persons with a disability. Indeed, the culture of persons with a disability also has an expressed preferred mode of reference—that is, "person-first language" in which one refers to a "person with a disability" rather than a "disabled person." Wright (1959) established a foundation for recognition of persons with a disability as a culturally identifiable group within which there are many individuals with varying characteristics.

Rehabilitation psychologists should be familiar with the work of Olkin (1999), who provides a thorough description of the cultural aspects of disability. Olkin, a psychologist with a disability, provides excellent insight into various aspects of the lives of persons with a disability: family life, sexuality and dating, testing, working, teaching, and more. Olkin employs humor as well as a forthright style in discussing topics that many might find awkward to confront. She characterizes herself as bicultural—living in the nondisabled world as well as the disability community. She describes the perspective of her peers as viewing people without disabilities as ABs (able-bodied) or TABs (temporarily able-bodied) and points out the cultural perspective of those without a disability as *non*disabled (emphasis hers). Appreciating that perspective, at once humorous and quite accurate, can assist a rehabilitation psychologist in starting to understand the cultural differences that can exist for persons with a disability.

One effective method of working with individuals in rehabilitation psychology involves recognizing the individual and cultural aspects of their lives and helping them establish a perspective, understanding, and meaning to their current (often acutely changed) life—the "new normal." This is an avenue to provide meaning, a critical aspect of individual identity as well as culture. It is not uncommon to hear the work of Frankl (2006) brought up in rehabilitation settings. Frankl, a concentration camp survivor, wrote of finding meaning in suffering, moving on in life, and personally growing from the process of doing so. Interested readers should review the thoughtful paper by Keany and Glueckauf (1993), which discusses some types of adaptive value change including enlarging the range of one's values and de-emphasizing physical prowess in favor of more cerebral pursuits. Some such modifications may be alien to the individual's culture, requiring much support and education of both the patient and the family.

Gusman and colleagues (1996) described what they referred to as a constructivist and developmental perspective using a "three-way mirror" reflecting the pretrauma, trauma, and posttrauma experience of the individual. They write of a "disorder of the multicultural self" in reference to difficulties with integrating the traumatic experience into one's self-identity as well as difficulty reintegrating the self into society.

Thus, the rehabilitation psychologist must consider not only multicultural and diversity issues with respect to gender, age, race, sexual orientation, nationality, religion, and other variables but also the additional factor of how the patient's cultural background and individual experience interact with disability. Although clearly not exhaustive, these brief examples provide the reader a sampling of the wide array of cultural, group, and other differences that make consideration of diversity issues paramount in everyday practice of rehabilitation psychology.

FOUR

Interpersonal Interaction

The relationship variable is doubtless one of the most frequently studied elements within human services, and the results are astoundingly robust. "No other treatment process variable has been so meticulously researched. A database check using 'therapeutic alliance' as the key search term produced 3,350 citations of books and articles" (J. C. Thomas & Hersen, 2010, p. 123). Sometimes called the "therapeutic alliance" or "working alliance," it has been shown to be a reliable predictor of therapy outcome—indeed, perhaps the primary such factor (Horvath & Bedi, 2002). The rehabilitation psychologist may not invariably be engaged in conventional "therapy" per se, but the expectation remains of creating and working within a therapeutic framework no less than in intensive psychotherapy or any other therapeutic milieu. Establishing rapport is essential—not only with the client/patient but also with the team, family members, ancillary staff, and organizational administration. This competency is an integral component that crosses all rehabilitation competencies.

The Relationship

The various approaches and schools of thought within psychological services that conceptualize the basic elements of the professional relationship share common foundational expectations. For our purposes we shall rely most heavily upon the work of the American Psychological Association (APA), the National Council of Schools and Programs of Professional Psychology (NCSPP), and the documents of the American Board of Rehabilitation Psychology (ABRP). The APA is the primary source for ethical principles and code of conduct, as well as establishment of core competencies. The NCSPP has provided important input regarding competencies expected in a professional psychology curriculum (Peterson et al., 1991). The ABRP has defined the competencies required for board certification in rehabilitation psychology. The ABRP literature is particularly beneficial for a student (and program) to address early on in the training experience, so as to understand the quality of acquired professional experience, knowledge, and skills for the highest level of professional recognition in rehabilitation psychology.

Competency in interpersonal interactions, as defined by the American Board of Rehabilitation Psychology (2011), requires that rehabilitation psychologists be sensitive to the welfare of others and respect their rights and dignity. They relate with empathy to patients and others, including treatment team members, striving to increase effectiveness in service provision. Finally, rehabilitation psychologists maintain requisite boundaries and are aware of the effect that their interactions may have on others.

Ethical Considerations

Attention is called to the American Psychological Association "Ethical Principles of Psychologists and Code of Conduct" (2002, 2010a), revised and updated from time to time, reflecting changes in legal, cultural, educational, and other aspects of the practice of professional psychology. The entire document is pertinent and should be familiar to every clinician, but several areas emphasize interpersonal interaction aspects. For example, Principle E, Respect for People's Rights and Dignity, states:

> Psychologists respect the dignity and worth of all people, and the rights of individuals to privacy, confidentiality, and self-determination. Psychologists are aware that special safeguards may be necessary to protect the rights and welfare of persons or communities whose vulnerabilities impair autonomous decision making. Psychologists are aware of and respect cultural, individual, and role differences, including those based on age, gender, gender identity, race, ethnicity, culture, national origin, religion, sexual orientation, disability, language, and socioeconomic status and consider these factors when working with members of such groups. Psychologists try to eliminate the effect on their work of biases based on those factors, and they do not knowingly participate in or condone activities of others based upon such prejudices (APA, 2010a).

Empathy

Empathy is doubtless a key component of professional psychology competence. Rehabilitation psychologists, in particular, should cultivate the ability to empathically interact with others so as to foster cohesive and effective treatment team functioning. The key words are *empathically* and *effective*.

We must keep in mind the difference between empathy and sympathy. It is easy to become overidentified with others' problems, particularly in rehabilitation settings where one deals on a daily basis with individuals whose lives have been drastically changed in multiple ways by injury or illness; such encounters may provoke strong self-referential emotions that can undercut one's objectivity. Although the two emotions share commonalities, they differ significantly. *Empathy* is "the intellectual identification with or vicarious experiencing of the feelings, thoughts, or attitudes of another," whereas *sympathy* is "the harmony or agreement in feeling, as between persons or on the part of one person with respect to another" (Webster's Collegiate Dictionary, 1996).

Unfortunately, the dictionary definition of empathy suggests a detached, cerebral function. The primary difference is the word *vicarious*, which means to exercise, receive, or suffer *in the place* of another. Understanding, compassion, care, and sharing of emotions are expected of the competent rehabilitation psychologist, coupled with avoidance of overidentification with the patient's concerns, pains, and challenges. Assisting, helping, encouraging, and even "feeling with" the patient must not preclude maintaining clinical objectivity.

Yet, rehabilitation psychologists must with specific intent attempt to understand the unseen and unheard pains and challenges of those with whom they work. Knowledge of others is a key component of differentiating self from others, thus allowing one to avoid many of the pitfalls spoken of in this and other chapters of this book. In fact, the *Core Curriculum in Professional Psychology* states: "The well-trained psychologist does not attempt to work with others without first gaining some knowledge of the larger context in which the client functions" (Polite & Bourg, 1991). The line between sympathy and empathy cannot be maintained without this knowledge and the continual effort to acknowledge it.

Awareness of Self and Others

Competence in interpersonal interactions means having a deep awareness of how you affect others and how others affect you. Awareness may seem to be a simple concept, but those who have personal experience with psychotherapy know the depth and breadth of what is required to "know yourself." Self-awareness can also be promoted by the experience of a personal emotional or physical challenge.

The concept of awareness is partially intellectual but more basically is experiential. Few psychological specialties can rival rehabilitation psychology in the demands placed on awareness of the complexities of interpersonal interactions and the difficulties of applying that knowledge to dealings with individuals who are partially paralyzed, in intense pain, or coping with sensory impairment. In these situations, the psychologist may learn more from the patient than the patient learns from the therapist.

Few training programs require personal psychotherapy, leaving the emerging psychologist to obtain self-knowledge through self-initiative. Nothing, however, takes the place of guidance and feedback from a well-seasoned senior psychologist mentor, regardless of one's own years of personal experience and training. Knowing how we perceive ourselves allows for establishing the professional parameters with other professionals and with patients. The patient's perception of "doctor" is often very different from that of the doctor himself or herself. Issues of authority, respect, and even admiration come into play, interacting with transference and countertransference, as well as compliance, cooperation, and attitude from and toward patients, staff, and colleagues.

Multicultural Factors

Although diversity is dealt with in more detail in other chapters, it is necessary to underscore the interpersonal aspects of multicultural differences. Issues of this sort may go unrecognized due to embedded prejudices and beliefs, both of the psychologist and of the client. Interpersonal relationships are often hindered by such beliefs, and problems or conflicts become mislabeled as noncompliance, resistance, apathy, or hostility. As observed by one expert, "…multicultural differences both energize the relationship as well as contribute to misunderstandings" (Campbell, 2006, p. 220).

General Human Relations

The APA Ethics Code sets forth Standard 3 as a broad yet detailed code in reference to human relations for all professional psychologists. It includes such items as unfair discrimination, sexual harassment, other harassment, avoiding harm, multiple relationships, conflicts of interest, third-party requests for services, exploitative relationships, cooperation with other professionals, informed consent, confidentiality, and a wide array of other potential issues that impinge upon one's interpersonal relations as they relate to professional behavior and practice.

Interpersonal Relationships and Stress

The rehabilitation psychologist is subjected to numerous and unique stress factors. Those with even the normal amount of empathy are apt from time to time to take on the emotional burdens of patients who endure exhausting and distressing physical and mental challenges. The urge to "help" is never far away, even when it is best to let patients learn and grow by struggling through on their own. Unpredicted emergencies, setbacks, medical complications, financial disappointments for help with a patient's special needs, the family's lack of support, and institutional realignments—all these and much more bring stress to the psychologist. Competency entails an awareness of one's own stress level and the utilization of stress reduction and management strategies.

Boundaries

There are two major aspects to be discussed concerning boundaries: (a) boundaries between the psychologist and other team members, supervisors, and professionals from other disciplines and (b) those between the psychologist and client (patient and/or family members). One type of professional boundary has to do with direct clinical services, whereas the other pertains more to administration and consultation.

Not all professional disciplines share the same code of conduct. That of the psychologist is one of the more prescriptive, proscriptive, and explicit. It is important to recognize the differences, and while respecting them, to adhere to what is expected from professional psychologists. One needs to be aware of the potential for interpersonal conflict due to differing ethical expectations of various other professional practitioners.

Also, it is important to recognize the difference between a psychologist in the consulting role (particularly organizational/business practice), where one might take a client to lunch or mutually enjoy a social event; for psychologists such would not be permissible. The nature of "dual relationships" and "conflicts of interest" must be assessed carefully and avoided.

Individual practice allows for a different style of professionalism than group practice might. The dictates of the group often superimpose sanctions, practice models, theories of management, and so forth upon the practitioner. Those who choose to practice within a group are accountable for all standards of professional conduct and appropriate interpersonal relations, regardless of the group philosophy. A "group dictate" or "group practice" is no excuse for unethical conduct.

Boundaries can also be blurred by financial donations, requirements and expectations (spoken and unspoken) of funding organizations, and spoken or unspoken expectations related to accepting gifts. Even the use of legitimate grants and research funds must be assessed carefully to ensure adherence to professional standards, as boundaries may be crossed (or, at least, temptations may arise) when seeking funding.

Boundaries and Sexual Behavior

Much has been written, and presumably much has been and is being taught, in current curricula regarding this topic. However, the focus is generally on the need for boundaries only within the *overt* sexual realm. Although this area needs specific and pronounced emphasis, other related matters merit attention as well: touching of any sort; visual transgressions; verbal transgressions, including references to body parts, bodily functions, sexual innuendos, and jokes or other questionable humorous conversation; physical gestures; and the invading of one's personal space. It is also possible to overstep one's boundaries by pushing for information of a personal nature too soon in the relationship and aggressively pursuing information that is being withheld by the patient. The astute psychologist knows where the boundaries are and senses when they are in danger of being violated. The APA Ethics Code is very specific in regard to behavior that may be interpreted as sexual harassment.

The rehabilitation psychologist is often (by default) seen as the staff member responsible for discussing issues of sexuality. In so doing, one must be alert for indications of patient resistance or disinterest (signs that the subject may have been prematurely broached) or, contrariwise, emergence of boundary-crossing flirtatiousness. Maintenance of professional distance is mandatory.

Other Harassment

Harassment is often defined by the subjectivity of another who is offended by unwanted behavior. Competent psychologists are attuned to the possibility that their actions and/or words may be offensive to others who hold different views. Factors such as age, gender, religion, sexual orientation, and culture are areas in which sensitivity to others is paramount, and in which insensitivity may lead to a perception of harassment.

Electronic Communication

The era of telecommunications brings a new element into interpersonal relations. E-mail and text messages tend to be cryptic, vague, ambiguous, and even rude. Special care must be taken with electronic etiquette as well as the assurance of confidentiality and security of information. Assumptions can be made and deleteriously acted upon, without informed consent, unintentionally, without the cooperation of the team and/or the patient, and often in disagreement with a previously agreed-upon treatment plan. Those who engage in treatment via electronic technology are encouraged to ruminate deeply on the particular challenges to interpersonal relationships via those media.

Educational and Training Program Standards

The *Core Curriculum in Professional Psychology* elucidates very clearly relational, interpersonal expectations. It emphasizes the knowledge of self, knowledge of others, skills, and attitudes. Knowledge of self includes awareness of our motivations, limitations, and peculiarities that may hinder or foster our ability to relate to others and therefore to become "therapeutic." "The role of self-knowledge in establishing effective professional relationships cuts across theoretical orientations. From a psychodynamic perspective, self-knowledge is critical in dealing effectively with transference and counter-transference issues" (Polite & Bourg, 1991, pp. 85–86).

Training programs do not always address the entire gamut of interpersonal relationships. Much is left to self-discovery, which sometimes occurs *after* damage is done. Included in such knowledge are individual *normal* personality differences, gender differences, lifestyle differences, cultural backgrounds, religious systems, and language barriers. Much emphasis is placed upon the *abnormal*, yet except for the pathology involved, rehabilitation psychologists observe and deal with that which is normal—or at least "unexceptional"—much of the time. There is a need for knowledge of the cognitive functioning of the patient, including the means of emotional expression employed by the patient in as many situations as possible, and the assumption that—unless and until proven otherwise—such is normal. The thinking and behavior may be both normal premorbidly and normal within the given disability experiences. Because all individuals live within both a microsystem and a macrosystem, oftentimes work orientations and even political elements become enmeshed in the process of problem solving and decision making.

The skill sets required for effective interpersonal interactions include the ability to communicate adequately and effectively, to engage others and effectively bring an end to a therapeutic relationship/environment, to establish and maintain rapport, and to at all times establish and maintain both therapist and patient dignity.

Attitude

Although "attitude" may be subsumed under many other topics, it bears individual importance for discussion. The centrality of interpersonal interactions requires competency in attitude. Because attitudes are built so concretely on values, a practicing psychologist will constantly be evaluating personal values and the integrity of their application. Polite and Bourg (1991, p. 87) indicate that the resultant attitudes are listed by the National Council of Schools and Programs in Professional Psychology as:

a. Intellectual curiosity and flexibility
b. Scientific skepticism
c. Open-mindedness
d. Psychological health
e. Belief in the capacity for change in human attitudes and behaviors
f. Appreciation of individual and cultural diversity
g. Interest in providing human services
h. Personal integrity and honesty
i. Capacity for developing interpersonal skills (typically, respect for others, personal relatedness)
j. Self-awareness

In summary, understanding and adhering to the basic principles for interpersonal relationships can *make* or *break* the rehabilitation psychologist. Often assumed to be understood, and thus at times relatively neglected in training programs, skill in and knowledge about interpersonal relationships are integral and essential competencies and an important part of the examination for board certification as a rehabilitation psychologist.

FIVE

Professional Identity

The professional identity of a rehabilitation psychologist evolves over the years, from early training to participation in lifelong learning activities, as well as in "giving back" to the field. In the view of the American Board of Rehabilitation Psychology (ABRP), the following are expected of successful candidates for board certification in the specialty area:

1. Actively participates in professional activities relevant to rehabilitation psychology
2. Has awareness of current issues facing the profession and implications of these issues for functioning as a rehabilitation psychologist
3. Seeks and utilizes consultation/supervision when needed or appropriate
4. Pursues continuing professional education commensurate with licensing requirements and professional development in specialty of rehabilitation psychology including continuing education (CE) in the area of rehabilitation psychology in the last 2 years (ABRP, 2011)

Many psychologists gain exposure to rehabilitation psychology to a greater or lesser degree over the course of their professional development and career. It would be unusual for a psychologist practicing with clinical populations not to have some involvement with persons with a disability at one time or another. However, the practice of rehabilitation psychology extends well beyond occasional exposure. Professional identity as a rehabilitation psychologist involves a developmental process that usually does not cohere until the postdoctoral years.

Professional identification as a rehabilitation psychologist includes many components, some more essential than others. The generic requirements of the profession include doctoral training in psychology and licensure at the independent doctoral level, followed by additional specialty-specific education, training, and experience. Continuing education in the specialty area of rehabilitation psychology, involvement with rehabilitation-related professional groups such as the American Psychological Association (APA) Division of Rehabilitation Psychology (Division 22), and attendance at relevant workshops and conferences are all aspects of establishing a professional identity as a rehabilitation psychologist. Increasingly, board certification in rehabilitation psychology through the ABRP is becoming expected of those identifying as rehabilitation psychologists. "Although ABPP [American Board of Professional Psychology] status is not the only manner of having an illustrious career in professional psychology, it is widely recognized and is directly tied to the practice of professional psychology" (Graham & Kim, 2011, p. 342).

Education and Training

Professional identity in rehabilitation psychology may start to become established for a given individual at any point in one's studies; however, doctoral preparation is the minimal level of training expected of rehabilitation psychologists. Although there are terminal master's degree programs in psychology, the field considers the doctoral degree to be the entrée into the profession. The APA holds to this stance, as do all but a very few jurisdictional licensing agencies. Board certification in the specialty area of rehabilitation psychology through the ABPP requires completion of doctoral training in psychology and licensure at the independent, doctoral level of practice, as well as further postdoctoral training/experience.

No single avenue is "the" way toward competence as a rehabilitation psychologist (see the exchange between K. R. Thomas & Chan, 2000, and Wegener, Elliott, & Hagglund, 2000). Parker and Chan (1990) pointed out that predoctoral training of rehabilitation psychologists was, at that time, rather generic and typically grew from experience in traditional clinical or counseling psychology assessment and intervention.

Historically, rehabilitation psychologists emerged from programs in clinical psychology, counseling psychology, school psychology, neuropsychology, and health psychology. Given that many, if not most, psychology graduates are now trained in doctoral programs accredited by the APA, and recognizing that the APA presently has only accredited clinical, counseling, and school psychology programs, the most recently trained rehabilitation psychologists likely have matriculated through a program in one of those three areas. As of this writing, a group of rehabilitation psychology training directors and educators are working to establish common and agreed-upon training and education guidelines to assist in more clearly defining such a preferred path (Stiers, Barisa, et al., in press; Stiers, Hanson, et al., 2012).

According to Glueckauf (2000), courses covering areas relevant to rehabilitation psychology (e.g., health psychology, geropsychology, neuropsychology) are found in many clinical and counseling doctoral programs. Pertinent training experiences also exist in internship and postdoctoral settings. The APA is now accrediting specialized postdoctoral fellowships in rehabilitation psychology. Ultimately, psychologists who choose to specialize in rehabilitation psychology are likely to seek specialty training through such programs as they increase in number and as the formal specialty training and experience guidelines are established and implemented.

It is unclear what percentage of practicum sites provide clinical experiences specifically focused on *rehabilitation*. Lewis, Hatcher, and Pate (2005) reported that 35% of practicum sites are located in hospital settings, medical centers, military hospitals, Veterans Administration hospitals, and private and state psychiatric settings; these are the types of facilities in which exposure to rehabilitation is likely to be at least a part of the experience. Cox et al. (2010) indicated that although current specialized doctoral training programs may be relatively small in number, there appears to be growth in the area, particularly when one reviews the number of internship and postdoctoral sites for training in rehabilitation psychology. Typically, initial exposure to rehabilitation psychology principles and practices does not happen during practica, but rather during internship or postdoctoral training.

An increase is evident in the number of APA-approved internships offering rehabilitation rotations in stroke, traumatic brain injury, renal dialysis, and pain units, as well as an increase in these programs in hospital settings. Glueckauf (2000) reported that 19 internship programs focusing on rehabilitation psychology were identified on the Division 22 website (http://www.div22.org/edu_train.php), and the more recent paper by Cox et al. (2010) reported a quadrupling of such programs. Psychology trainees are exposed to rehabilitation assessments and interventions as well as the multidisciplinary team approach in such settings (Glueckauf, 2000).

Patterson and Hanson (1995) reported that it is at the postdoctoral level where systematic and comprehensive training in rehabilitation psychology occurs. Patterson (1997) identified 19 postdoctoral programs that offered broad-based training in rehabilitation psychology. The posted listing of programs on the Division 22 website changes, and therefore the numbers may vary as new programs are added (or others deleted): Cox et al. (2010) reported 28 programs, Hibbard and Cox (2010) reported 32, and a recent review of the number of postdoctoral training sites listed found 43—further indication of the growth of opportunities in rehabilitation psychology training over the past decade (http://www.div22.org/edu_train.php). As more programs seek APA accreditation, successful completion of a rehabilitation psychology postdoctoral training program will likely become the expectation in the field rather than the exception. Specialized postdoctoral training in rehabilitation psychology will also serve as one type of evidence of competency as an advanced clinician in the area of rehabilitation psychology.

Areas of Focus Within the Specialty

There is a tremendous range of conditions and disabilities addressed by rehabilitation psychologists, and practitioners utilize clinical skills from prior training and experience in a variety of areas. These may include clinical and counseling psychology, developmental psychology, school psychology, educational psychology, neuropsychology, social psychology, medical psychology, health psychology, knowledge of individual and family systems, and community/public health policy (Hibbard & Cox, 2010).

As rehabilitation psychologists (and/or those in training) gain experience, they often develop particular interest in areas within the larger field of rehabilitation psychology. Many, perhaps most, rehabilitation psychologists eventually self-identify areas of interest in which they specialize. They may focus on childhood and developmental issues that include asthma, attention deficit hyperactivity disorder, cerebral palsy, childhood diabetes, and learning disorders. Such practitioners typically are closely involved with educational systems and family systems. Other rehabilitation psychologists focus on conditions such as stroke, dementia, cardiovascular disease, and degenerative disc disease that tend to affect older populations. There are also those who are involved more with specific diagnostic entities or syndromes that are not so age related (e.g., spinal cord injury, brain injury, burns), treating patients of all ages. Involvement with particular diagnoses is often also associated with participation in local or national organizations associated with that area (e.g., many who work in brain injury rehabilitation are members of a state or national Brain Injury Association).

Regardless of an individual rehabilitation psychologist's area of focus, his or her practice includes disability-related issues in assessment, intervention, and consultation. Also, the practice incorporates evaluation and treatment of individuals with disabling conditions as part of a larger system, and this is an integral concept in the specialty. An understanding of and an ability to work collaboratively with the variety of professional disciplines that contribute to rehabilitation are essential aspects of a rehabilitation psychologist's work and are central to one's identification with the specialty. Such work requires multifaceted knowledge and skills, and assessment of competence in rehabilitation psychology is of necessity complex and multifactorial.

Board Certification

Professionals and consumers alike have sought to identify competent psychologists within specialty areas. Public accountability and a public demand for identification of specialty competence have been cited as major reasons for the need to articulate what defines competency in specialty areas (Rodolfa et al., 2005). Areas of specialty practice in psychology have been defined by the APA, the Council of Specialties in Professional Psychology (CoS), and the ABPP. The ABPP is the only entity among them that not only addresses the concept of specialty as an area of practice but also credentials *individual psychologists* as specialists. Rodolfa et al. (2005) noted that the ABPP is the only organization that uses the term *competency* in its definition.

It is quite reasonable to expect competence to be a core characteristic of a profession. Medicine, law, and psychology are among the professions that have established methods to recognize competence. The APA "Ethical Principles of Psychologists and Code of Conduct" (2002), in addressing consumer protection, states that one should practice within one's area of competence.

Arising out of this focus on competency, consumer protection, and professional responsibility is a movement toward widespread board certification, as this can serve as one means of assessing competency to practice in a given psychological specialty. Competence in rehabilitation psychology is assessed and recognized through the board certification process of the American Board of Rehabilitation Psychology, a member board of the American Board of Professional Psychology http://www.abpp.org/i4a/pages/index.cfm?pageid=3363). A primary purpose of the ABPP's board certification process is protecting the public by certifying specialists through competency-based examinations.

Increasingly, the granting of hospital and staff privileges requires board certification. Some hospitals already require that psychologists on staff be board certified, just as are the physicians on staff. For the past 10 to 15 years, any psychologist hired within the Department of Psychiatry and Psychology of the Mayo Clinic is expected to obtain ABPP board certification in their chosen field of expertise (Rohe, personal communication, January 10, 2008).

Involvement: Association Membership, Conferences, and Continuing Education

The primary organization to which most rehabilitation psychologists belong is the American Psychological Association's Division of Rehabilitation Psychology (Division 22). Another is the American Congress of Rehabilitation Medicine (ACRM). Many also belong to organizations that focus on specific diagnostic or disability areas such as the Brain Injury Association of America (BIAA), American Cancer Society, Multiple Sclerosis Society, and others.

The field of psychology does not lie dormant; therefore, psychologists are expected to engage in lifelong learning in order to provide the best clinical services based on the most recent science. As of this writing, ABPP is formulating plans for a "maintenance of competence" process in which each specialty board will establish guidelines for periodic demonstration by its members that they have kept current with advances in their particular specialty. Continuing education activities such as workshops, conferences, reading current journal articles (for which one may earn CE credits), and active membership in rehabilitation-related associations and organizations can serve to keep rehabilitation psychologists up-to-date with advances in the specialty area. Active participation—as a learner as well as a teacher—can provide evidence of one's commitment to the specialty. The annual Division 22/ABRP midyear conference, a joint effort of the two organizations for more than 10 years, provides educational opportunities as well an outstanding venue within which rehabilitation psychologists may interact with others of like interests.

In addition, rehabilitation psychologists in academic, health care, and other large organizational settings may advance professional identity by providing educational and training opportunities to the next generation of rehabilitation psychologists. Although continuing education is perhaps more readily conducted in these settings, there are other avenues as well—mentoring individuals and even providing clinical supervision in independent practices can provide additional opportunity for rehabilitation psychologists to foster their own professional growth as well as that of others and the field at large.

PART III

Functional Competencies

SIX

Assessment

Although the name of the specialty emphasizes treatment, effective rehabilitation psychology interventions derive from comprehensive and accurate assessment of the multiple neurobehavioral, psychosocial, and environmental factors with which persons with disabilities and their families must grapple. This complex enterprise encompasses both science-based practice and interpretive art. These dovetailing processes entail review of available records, a thorough clinical interview with the patient (as permitted by his or her cognitive and physical condition), discussions with informed collaterals, formal testing with standardized instruments, nonstandard assessment when deemed useful, behavioral observations (in both one-on-one interactions and larger social settings), analysis of test results with full recognition of potential performance-limiting factors, and extraction of therapeutically relevant information from the obtained facts, figures, and impressions.

Because of the prominence of assessment skills in rehabilitation psychology, every specific "assessment competency" that is listed by the American Board of Rehabilitation Psychology (ABRP) as relevant to the field is viewed as "essential," the sole domain in which every item is so designated. Thus, to achieve board certification, candidates must demonstrate specialist-level skills in evaluation across many medical conditions employing a range of procedures in a sensible and defensible manner.

The assessment process in rehabilitation psychology might best be construed as a mosaic composed of pieces from several other specialties embedded among many that are unique to the specialty of rehabilitation psychology. This reflects the multifaceted knowledge and skills that psychologists working in rehabilitation settings must acquire and refine. Just as rehabilitation physicians need a good grasp of (at a minimum) internal medicine, neurology, orthopedics, psychiatry, and pharmacology, so, too, must rehabilitation psychologists be familiar with concepts and tools primarily associated with health psychology, clinical psychology, educational psychology, social psychology, and neuropsychology in addition to an evolving core corpus of rehabilitation psychology–specific facts and measures. Reid-Arndt et al. (2010) encapsulated the activities of rehabilitation psychology as follows:

> Drawing on expertise in functional neuroanatomy, psychometric theory, psychopathology, psychosocial models of illness and disability, and psychological and neuropsychological assessment and treatment applications, rehabilitation psychologists provide essential assessment services in both inpatient and outpatient settings. Recognizing the multiple determinants of patient outcomes, rehabilitation psychologists take a multifactorial, multidimensional approach to assessment of cognitive functions, emotional state, behavior, personality, family dynamics, and the environment to which the patient will ultimately return (p. 66).

The last of these requires attention to the patient's ability to deal with social and cultural "handicapping" forces such as negative attitudes, opinions, comments, and even overt behaviors of the portion of the public that is ill-informed about (or frightened by) disability, as well as the ever-present environmental challenges for persons who must cope with a world architecturally designed for those without physical, cognitive, or sensory limitations.

Before considering some specific assessment skills required of a rehabilitation psychologist, some general discussion of the nature and history of psychological assessment is in order. While assessment was, for many years, a fundamental and relatively unique skill offered by psychologists, the proportion of time devoted to assessment declined from the late 1950s to the 1970s (e.g., Lubin & Lubin, 1972; Lubin, Lubin, Matarazzo, & Seever, 1986), perhaps because more professional time was being spent providing psychotherapy (Gold & De Piano, 1992). Nonetheless, assessment remained an essential component of the psychologist's armamentarium, although perhaps in a new form, replacing what Gold and De Piano called the "increasingly outmoded model" of assessment as involving "testing of an individual person conducted as a prelude to treatment for the primary purpose of formulating a diagnosis" (p. 91). In the view of these authors, the criteria-based diagnostic schemes in the *Diagnostic and Statistical Manual of Mental Disorders* were better served through observation and interview than formal testing.

Two decades ago, Gold and De Piano (1992) made several observations about assessment that are highly pertinent to the practice of rehabilitation psychology. First, they pointed out the importance of consultative skills in the assessment process, as one must clarify with the referring source just what is being requested; frequent consultation (discussed in more detail in Chapter 7) is an essential aspect of the rehabilitation psychologist's daily life, given that he or she often operates as a member of a treating team (Butt & Caplan, 2010). Of course, consultations are also carried out for purposes beyond assessment including management of problem behaviors, coordination of treatment of chronic pain, school and community re-entry, and vocational restoration.

Gold and De Piano also noted that assessment skills should be applied to measurement of outcomes, an important contemporary function of rehabilitation psychologists (McAweeney & Crewe, 2000). Gold and De Piano further argued for the importance of a solid grasp of the conceptual underpinnings of the assessment process and familiarity with supporting science, without which the psychologist would be little more than a technician (see the science base chapter 10 in this text for discussion of some of the evidentiary core of the field). In addition, these authors wrote of the importance of converting test scores into interpretations. "The psychologist must be able to translate findings into jargon-free terminology" (p. 94) that can be understood by examinees and referral sources; a logical corollary is the importance of the further translation of interpretations into statements about likely impact on function, broadly construed. They also noted that it is frequently of greatest importance to identify patient strengths rather than deficits, as these can lead to evidence-based suggestions about treatment. This is clearly the historical modus operandi of the rehabilitation psychologist (Caplan, 1982).

As argued by Gold and De Piano, "assessment" does not equal "testing." Furthermore: "Assessment is an ongoing, interactive and inclusive process that serves to describe, conceptualize, characterize, and predict relevant aspects of a client" (Bent, 1992, p. 78), to which one might add by way of emphasis "to achieve a multidimensional *understanding of* the client— his or her problems, assets, concerns, goals, and plans," not merely assign a diagnosis. Testing constitutes one useful source of data, the results of which must be integrated with information gleaned from interviews with patients and other informed sources such as family and friends, observations of behavior, review of records, and consultations with other treating clinicians. The multidisciplinary team structure that is historically typical of the rehabilitation setting provides opportunities for the rehabilitation psychologist to gather input from all of these sources with the aim of developing a broad understanding of the given patient's psychological and neuropsychological status; primary roles in the family, workplace, and community; grasp of his or her condition and prognosis; hopes and expectations for both the rehabilitation process and postdischarge life; and resources (of all types) available to assist him or her in grappling with the facts and implications of disability.

The theoretical roots of rehabilitation psychology lie in social psychological concepts about interaction between person and environment (D. Dunn, 2010), a harbinger of the now widely accepted biopsychosocial model of illness. This expansive view of the multiple determinants of behavior dictates broad-based assessment of the many factors that can affect an individual's accommodation to new-onset or congenital disability. Furthermore, rehabilitation psychologists often work with their clients both during hospitalization and after discharge, and the relevance of various factors can differ between the two phases. Consequently, rehabilitation psychologists have historically been well aware of the need to consider in their evaluations not only the personality, emotional response to illness, and coping strategies of the person with a disability but also the impact of family members (Chwalisz & Dollinger, 2010), friends, members of the treatment team (Caplan & Reidy, 1996) educational and vocational factors (Wade & Walz, 2010), accessibility in the community, and even the prevailing political zeitgeist as it affects health care policy (Ashkenazi, Hagglund, Lee, & Swaine, 2010).

Rehabilitation psychologists generally accept the emphasis in rehabilitation medicine on "function," a term that can connote (as in the International Classification of Functioning, Disability and Health scheme) the activity of a specific organ (e.g., kidney) or body part (e.g., arm) or a "real world" action such as walking or cooking. A related concept, also heavily emphasized in rehabilitation, is "quality of life," defined by Heinemann and Mallinson (2010) as "...individuals' perceptions of their health in relation to their expectations" (p. 147).

Adherence to the importance of these notions dictates that assessment in rehabilitation psychology should assist the treating team in devising interventions that will improve function and enhance quality of life consistent with the individual's preferences. In this way, rehabilitation neuropsychological assessment has long differed from traditional diagnostic neuropsychological practice—that is, simply documenting deficits in cognition, attention, memory, perception, and so forth is not sufficient; rather, the rehabilitation clinician must draw inferences about (a) how identified deficits will likely affect functional activities and (a) how these can be remediated/ameliorated or their impact minimized. (NB: In recent years, the American Board of Clinical Neuropsychology has also urged that case study material submitted for review include recommendations for treatment derived from the test data.)

We now examine some domains of assessment identified as essential "functional competencies"—ones that must be demonstrated to earn board certification by the ABRP. These should be considered illustrative but not exhaustive, given space constraints. Furthermore, rehabilitation psychologists who work in certain settings (such as those focused on treatment of individuals with a particular condition such as severe burns or spinal cord injury) may find other assessment skills to be indispensable for their work.

Adjustment to Disability: Patient

Perhaps the most fundamental aim of rehabilitation psychology assessment is to understand how individuals with disabilities deal with their limitations on an emotional level and to assist them in exploiting preserved skills as they accommodate to the "new normal." Concepts from clinical psychology and health psychology such as "coping" and "resilience" (White, Driver, & Warren, 2008) are most pertinent in this effort (Johnson-Greene & Touradji, 2010). The explosion of "positive psychology" (Ehde, 2010) has been a welcome development, as it has renewed rehabilitation researchers' and clinicians' awareness of the historic emphasis on "ability, not disability." Although some might find it unthinkable that such could exist, positive consequences of acute-onset disabilities such as spinal cord injury or stroke have been identified (e.g., Ganstad, Norman, & Barton, 2009; Gillen, 2005; McMillen & Cook, 2003). A recent section of *Rehabilitation Psychology* (deRoon-Cassini, Mancini, Rusch, & Bonanno, 2010; Kortte, Gilbert, Gorman, & Wegener, 2010; Quale & Schanke, 2010; Seale, Berges, Ottenbacher, & Ostir, 2010; White, Driver, & Warren, 2010) consisted of five articles that provided considerable evidence of the facilitating effect on both functional and psychological outcome following traumatic injuries of positive psychological factors such as "resilience" and "positive emotions."

Elliott and Umlauf (1995) argued that rehabilitation psychology historically was "...characterized by a preoccupation with the level of distress in reaction to acquired disability" (p. 326). This was understandable, perhaps, at a time when "stage theories" of adjustment to stressful events (including disability) were widely accepted, and the "requirement of mourning" was imposed on individuals with newly acquired disability for whom depression was seen as an inevitable—indeed, necessary—reaction if "adjustment to disability" was ever to be achieved. The contemporary view holds that, although emotional reactions for which the "stages" were named (e.g., depression, denial) certainly may occur, it is a substantial oversimplification (as well as a disservice to all) to expect them to unfold in a predictable, invariant sequence (e.g., Caplan & Shechter, 1987; Elliott & Frank, 1996) and to infer that a problem exists if a particular patient presents otherwise. Furthermore, assessments by rehabilitation psychologists should encompass evaluation of both positive (e.g., resilience) and negative (e.g., chaotic family structure) influences, as both are relevant in formulation of treatment plans. This is a multimethod process that may include interviews, observations, testing, and consultations with other team members.

Detailed interviews are almost certainly the best source of information about the extent of patients' understanding of their condition and prognosis and the importance of participation in rehabilitation, their preferences for particular coping strategies or stress management tactics, and their expectations for posthospital life (see Table 14.1 in Rohe, 2010, for an invaluable list of information to be gleaned from the interview); all of these factors help shape the individual's emotional adjustment. The psychologist must attempt to distinguish between enduring personality characteristics (traits) and more transient reactions to illness/injury and hospitalization (states).

Traditional measures of mood may have a role, but interpretation must proceed carefully, due to the possibility of spurious or misleading findings. Experienced rehabilitation psychologists have long been aware (e.g., Myerson, 1957) that many, if not most, measures of psychological function were normed on physically healthy people, with the consequence that the various scales and indices derived therefrom may be misleading when applied uncritically to persons with disabilities. For example, certain items on psychodiagnostic instruments such as the Minnesota Multiphasic Personality Inventory-2 and Symptom Checkllist-90-R concern physical symptoms that are typical consequences of many disabling conditions (e.g., loss of bowel and bladder control in persons with quadriplegia).

Individuals with certain disabilities who answer such questions honestly may produce spuriously "pathological" profiles, as their endorsements carry very different diagnostic significance than they do for physically healthy people. Hence, the experienced rehabilitation psychologist has learned to look "beyond the information given" by index or summary scores, examining responses to individual items to minimize the chances of erroneous diagnosis and mislabeling (Caplan & Shechter, 1993).

Efforts have been devoted to identifying and eliminating potentially distorting items as a function of given diagnostic categories (e.g., Gass, 1992; Meyerink, Reitan, & Selz, 1988; Woessner & Caplan, 1995), but some (Stein, Sliwinski, Gordon, & Hibbard, 1996) have cautioned that important information may be lost thereby. The best approach, therefore, would appear to lie in maintaining awareness of the *possibility* (not inevitability) of spurious elevations and evaluating the multiple determinants of responses to discern whether, for example, a report of "sleep disruption" is a manifestation of depression or results from sleeping in an unfamiliar environment, being turned every 2 hours to prevent bedsores, or being paired with a snoring or otherwise disruptive neighbor.

Observation of patients on the rehabilitation unit or in physical therapy, speech therapy, and occupational therapy may offer clues to their mood, coping abilities, and understanding of their condition. Those who exhibit minimal motivation or outright resistance may be depressed or have limited awareness that progress in rehabilitation demands effort; indeed, the whole concept of "chronic illness" may be foreign to some (especially younger patients), who are accustomed to "sickness" being a temporary state. Important diagnostic data can be gathered by seeing how the individual responds when confronted with newly challenging tasks.

Adjustment to Disability: Family

The effects of disabling conditions extend to family members, and no assessment would be truly complete without information about how relatives understand the illness/injury and prognosis, their expectations for involvement in rehabilitation and in postdischarge care, and their views of possible or likely changes in family roles and responsibilities as a result of their loved one's disability (Shewchuck & Elliott, 2000). Just how—and how much—education and counseling are offered will depend on the psychologist's assessment of the family situation. As with patients themselves, in-depth interviews are probably the best avenue by which to obtain this information, but formal measures such as the McMaster Family

Assessment Device (Epstein, Baldwin, & Bishop, 1983) can be useful as well. In addition, standard measures of mood taken from the patient can also be used with relatives but without the same concerns about potentially spurious elevations of pathological indices.

In evaluating family adjustment, it is usually vital to establish just how well informed family members are about their loved one's condition. Inaccurate or incomplete information can lead to misunderstanding and misattribution, eventuating in suboptimal adjustment all around. For example, it is imperative that the wife of a cognitively impaired male stroke survivor receive adequate explanations of the nature of her husband's deficits and their neurological etiology. Being able to say to herself, "That's the stroke talking, not Bob" when her previously easygoing but now disinhibited husband lashes out at her can help to minimize the anger and stress she may feel in her new role as caregiver, thereby promoting her own adjustment and decreasing the likelihood of burnout. Given the significance of the caregiver's perceived burden for ultimate long-term outcome (Chwalisz & Dollinger, 2010), the effective rehabilitation psychologist recognizes the value of time devoted to family teaching. Education about previously foreign neurobehavioral phenomena like neglect, aprosodia, or aphasia can reduce the traumatic impact on relatives of their early confrontations with these behaviors. The skilled rehabilitation psychologist will, therefore, seek to uncover—and fill in—any important gaps in the family's grasp of relevant medical and neurobehavioral facts.

Identification of Extent and Nature of Disability and Preserved Abilities

"Ability, not disability" is a common theme in rehabilitation. By encouraging patients to maintain awareness of—and pride in—those skills and abilities that are unaffected by disability (or those that can now be cultivated), psychologists promote their patients' psychological balance and a better perspective on what they have lost and what remains. This effort was captured nicely in a question posed by one of the pioneers of rehabilitation psychology, Leonard Diller, PhD, to a depressed person with a recent spinal cord injury. Dr. Diller asked, "Aren't you more than someone who walks?" In this way, one can begin to elicit an inventory of preserved talents, interests, and aims, thereby creating a healthy—and realistic—counterweight to the understandably depressing mental set held by someone who had lost the ability to ambulate.

For the psychologist, it is especially vital to distinguish between "can do" and "does do," that is, to contrast "capability" with "performance" and to help identify influences that may prevent the latter from reaching the level of the former. Certain factors (often emotional ones) may foster good participation in physical therapy but lead to apparent inertia on the nursing unit. The author worked with one adolescent male with paraplegia who executed independent transfers skillfully in the therapy gym but resisted doing so from wheelchair back to bed. The difference? The gym appealed to his "macho" side, and he could show off a bit in front of others, but he saw it as the nurses' job to serve patients' needs, even if the "needs" were imaginary. Modest intervention, focusing on the importance of mastering transfers to and from various surfaces and establishing good routines in preparation for discharge, promoted independent transferring, regardless of location.

Educational and/or Vocational Capacities

As disability can arise at any age, the rehabilitation psychologist must be equipped to evaluate and advise concerning at least two categories of postrehabilitation productive activity—return to school and return to work. Clearly, the pertinent measures are quite different, but it is likely (although not essential) that evaluations for both purposes will take place during outpatient treatment. Assessments completed too early in the recovery process may merely document deficits that will diminish to some degree over time because of both natural recovery and the impact of treatment; predictive value will be limited. Thus, it is generally preferable to delay testing for the purposes of educational/vocational advice.

For those for whom return to school is anticipated, conventional measures of academic achievement (e.g., Wide Range Achievement Test-4, Woodcock-Johnson tests) are useful in determining whether these skills have been affected, especially if earlier school records can be made available. These will usually contain not only the individual's grades and class rank but also results of standardized tests given at regular intervals in most states. This information can provide a premorbid baseline against which one can compare current results to gauge whether cognitive loss has occurred and the extent of such decline.

Tests used in the course of neuropsychological evaluation (e.g., of attention, memory, and executive function) may offer insight into desirable accommodations that the school may need to put into place as required by the Americans With Disabilities Act (ADA). It should be considered an essential part of the assessment process to advise examinees (and their parents) about their rights to such accommodations under the ADA. In difficult economic times, school systems may be understandably reluctant to part with funds in such cases, so the conclusions and recommendations should be as specific and well supported as possible.

For those who desire to enter the workforce or for whom the formal educational path is not an option (e.g., because of lack of interest, acquired cognitive deficits, or some other reason), several of well-established vocational measures are available to help them crystallize their interests and skills (Fraser & Johnson, 2010). Rehabilitation psychology has a long historical connection with vocational rehabilitation; many early rehabilitation specialists viewed resumption of competitive employment as the "brass ring" of rehabilitation, and this is still a most meaningful goal for many rehabilitation patients (Vestling, Tufvesson, & Iwarsson, 2003).

An obvious distinction is that between vocational "interests" and "aptitudes." The large number of frustrated athletes and rock stars in the general population illustrates this difference. As Leahy (1995) pointed out, interests and aptitudes are positively correlated, but the relation is not perfect, so both factors must be evaluated. Common instruments for measuring vocational interests include the Kuder General Interest Survey and Kuder Occupational Interest Survey, Strong Interest Inventory, Wide Range Interest-Opinion Test, and Self-Directed Search. For measuring aptitude, one might employ the Differential Aptitude Test of General Aptitude Test Battery (see Leahy, 1995, for discussion). Interested readers should consult Power (2006) for a comprehensive discussion of measures and the process. Related to assessment of aptitudes is the evaluation of general cognitive abilities. Caplan and Shechter (1991) provided a useful overview of the value of neuropsychological assessment in vocational counseling.

In instances where the individual was previously employed, a thorough work history should be taken addressing specific responsibilities, limitations, results of performance evaluations, relations with coworkers, and reasons for leaving prior positions. It could be helpful to know whether any people with disabilities currently work at the site in question; if so, that might augur well for the employer's willingness to make accommodations. Also, information from physicians and therapists concerning matters such as strength, dexterity, and stamina should be integrated into the analysis. Often overlooked in this effort, but of considerable importance, is the impact of psychological factors on vocational readiness. As observed by Szymanski (2000), physical factors and limitations have obvious implications for work, but so does the patient's emotional state, whether the patient is depressed (with accompanying diminished motivation), anxious about community re-entry as a person with a disability, or fearful of reinjury (especially if the disability was acquired on the job).

Leahy (1995) also wisely noted the importance of ensuring that patients do not overgeneralize the effects of their disability on vocational options—that is, do not unnecessarily rule out certain possibilities on the (possibly unwarranted) assumption that these jobs are foreclosed to them because of their disability. Here, certainly, it is vital that patients understand their rights under both the ADA (most critically the mandate for "reasonable accommodations") and (if they were employed at the time of onset of illness or injury) the Family Medical Leave Act (see Wegener & Stiers, 2010, for discussion). In addition, the facilitating effect of various forms of assistive technology should be considered (Kirsch & Scherer, 2010).

The outcome of the assessment may point toward job training (or retraining); a supported work trial (Wehman et al., 1989), with or without accommodations (which could involve return to a prior position initially on a part-time basis or a supported work experience); delay while further recovery occurs or greater clarification of interests and aptitudes proceeds; or filing for disability benefits if return to work does not seem likely.

Personality and Emotional Functioning

Although linked in the ABRP scheme of competencies, assessment of these two phenomena differs in meaningful ways. The most fundamental distinction is that "personality" refers to enduring characteristics, whereas "emotions" can, of course, be transient; in the process of accommodating to disability, emotional state certainly can vary markedly and is more modifiable. On the other hand, some research suggests that personality tends to be altered little by new-onset disability (e.g., Hollick et al., 2001; Kurtz, Putnam, & Stone, 1998).

Understanding a patient's long-standing personality characteristics can offer some clues about how the individual will deal with disability and the process of rehabilitation. For example, Elliott et al. (1991) reported that those persons with spinal cord injury who displayed greater assertiveness in social settings exhibited less distress and better psychosocial functioning than those who were more passive. Another subject of recent investigation is spirituality, with the general finding being positive associations between existential spiritual orientation and quality of life (Albright, Forchheimer, & Tate, 2010). This remains a relatively untapped area from an empirical point of view but a rich one clinically, as the onset of disability can precipitate a spiritual crisis, prompting confrontation with one's mortality, disruption of the foundations of one's identity, and questioning of one's fundamental values.

There is some evidence of predisposing characteristics for certain rehabilitation-relevant conditions. For instance, persons who sustain traumatic brain injury (TBI) are more likely to have criminal records (Kreutzer, Marwitz, & Witol, 1996) or a history of learning disabilities or emotional problems (Woodward et al., 1999). For TBI and other types of traumatically acquired disabilities such as spinal cord injury, some early research suggested that injured individuals were premorbidly more likely to engage in risk-taking behaviors, in the course of which they were injured (e.g., Bourestom & Howard, 1965; Fordyce, 1964). Although the issue remains unsettled, a recent paper by Berry, Elliott, and Rivera (2007) using cluster analysis identified three personality prototypes among individuals with spinal cord injury, the most common being what they termed the "undercontrolled" variety, suggesting parallels with the impulsive risk takers discussed in earlier studies.

Assessment of both personality characteristics and emotional state in persons with disabilities must be done with caution, keeping in mind the caveats about possible misinterpretation discussed previously under the section Adjustment to Disability: Patient. As observed by Elliott and Umlauf (1995), "...inappropriate and insensitive use of psychological instruments with clientele limited in physical capacity can produce erroneous and misleading results and imprecise observations about the respondent" (p. 325). They noted the desirability of developing normative data sets for persons with disabilities, and indeed, some do exist. For example, there have been studies of both the Symptom Checklist-90 and its abbreviation, the Brief Symptom Inventory (BSI), with persons with spinal cord injury (Buckelew, Baumstark, Frank, & Hewett, 1994; Heinrich, Tate, & Buckelew, 1994). Heinrich et al. identified eight BSI symptoms (roughly 15% of the total) that were endorsed at high rates by persons with spinal cord injury, but these reflected actual physical and psychosocial consequences of the injury rather than emotional responses.

A welcome trend is evident in the use of what Radnitz, Bockian, and Moran (2000) called "non-pathology-based assessment of personality." They noted that instruments such as the Millon Behavioral Health Inventory (Millon, Green, & Meagher, 1982; now the Millon Behavioral Medicine Diagnostic, Millon, Antoni, Minor, & Grossman, 2006) and NEO-Personality Inventory (Costa & McCrae, 1992; now in its 3rd edition) yield information that goes beyond simple diagnosis, offering clues as to how best to work with the patient in rehabilitation.

Cognitive Abilities

Expertise in evaluating cognition is shared with many other psychological specialties, especially neuropsychology. The competent rehabilitation psychologist has a solid grasp of the neuropsychological consequences of common rehabilitation conditions such as stroke, TBI, and multiple sclerosis (Caplan, 2010; Chiaravalloti & DeLuca, 2010; Larson, Kirschner, Bode, Heinemann, Clorfene, & Goodman, 2003; Ricker & Rosenthal, 2010). Furthermore, given demographic trends supporting the "graying of America," familiarity with cognitive changes in normal and abnormal aging is expected (Lichtenberg & Schneider, 2010), as is awareness of common comorbidities (e.g., brain injury co-occurring with spinal cord injury) that may mandate testing of cognitive skills. As mentioned earlier, the rehabilitation psychologist's assessment of cognition should lead to suggestions about treatment and implications of observed deficits and retained skills for daily life functioning (Marcotte & Grant, 2010). Other specialties have in recent years recognized the importance of this "ecological leap" (given that the neuropsychological diagnostic task of identifying and localizing lesions essentially no longer exists), but it has been part and parcel of the rehabilitation psychologist's charge for at least 3 decades (Caplan, 1982).

In light of the ever-decreasing rehabilitation unit length of stay, as well as the competition among multiple specialties for patient time, the cognitive testing conducted by the rehabilitation psychologist will generally need to be focused and selective, guided by the most pressing referral questions. In this setting, the "flexible battery" or "hypothesis testing" approach tends to be the method of choice. (An exception involves testing of patients with multiple sclerosis, as a well-conceived brief battery has been developed; Benedict et al., 2002). Furthermore, because much of rehabilitation involves new learning (or relearning of old skills), testing of memory will likely be a vital and unique contribution of the rehabilitation psychologist's assessment. Also, given the salience of executive functions for functional outcome (e.g., Pohjasvaara et al., 2002), assessment of this domain will often be paramount. A similar point applies to visual-perceptual skills, as deficits in this area can have major implications for treatment progress and ultimate outcome (Gialanella & Mattioli, 1992).

One of the more distinctive features of assessment in rehabilitation psychology is the use of nonstandard procedures for evaluation of cognitive abilities via (a) modifications of existing tests and (b) development of novel measures (although this is also seen in the area of cognitive neuropsychology, where exquisitely detailed and innovatively assessed case studies are prevalent). Many individuals seen in rehabilitation settings have disabilities that can complicate conventional administration and interpretation of neuropsychological tests. For example, individuals with unilateral neglect may only "see" a portion of any visually administered test, earning low scores for that reason alone. Also, persons with high-level quadriplegia or severe visual impairment cannot be given most of the traditional Performance measures from the Wechsler scales (Wechsler 2008). Those with dominant hemiplegia are at some disadvantage on many tests that require manual responses if they must use the nonpreferred hand alone. However, it should be noted that some tasks such as the Trail Making Test (LoSasso, Rapport, Axelrod, & Reeder, 1998) or clock drawing (Bush, 2000) can be performed almost equally well with the nondominant hand.

Confronted on a daily basis with these kinds of clinical challenges, rehabilitation psychologists have endeavored to identify ways to alter traditional tests in minor ways to permit more valid assessment of the construct(s) that tests are intended to measure. For example, Berninger, Gans, St. James, and Connors (1988) developed response alternatives for each Verbal item and for the Picture Completion items on the Wechsler Adult Intelligence Scale-Revised. Examinees with speech deficits (e.g., from stroke or cerebral palsy) could point to their selections. Similarly, Schultheis, Caplan, Ricker, and Woessner (2000) created multiple choices for items on the Hooper Visual Organization Test, thus permitting its use with individuals with expressive language disorders. Caplan (1988) created a "midline" version (i.e., response choices arrayed in a single column instead of a 2 × 3 matrix) of the Raven Coloured Progressive Matrices for use with patients exhibiting unilateral neglect. This format eliminated the lateral scanning requirement, increasing the likelihood that these patients would actually see all response alternatives, not just those on the nonneglected side.

Other methods of "testing the limits" familiar to practitioners of other specialties that are most useful in rehabilitation settings include dispensing with time limits and allowing examinees with motor impairment or behavioral slowing to work to completion or photo-enlarging materials that a visually impaired individual must read or analyze. These procedural modifications may preclude use of available normative data, but there is a tradeoff in that the results may more accurately reflect the skills that the test purports to measure. The manual for the Wechsler Adult Intelligence

Scale-IV explicitly warns against "...attribut(ing) low performance on a cognitive test to low intellectual ability when, in fact, it may be related to physical, language or sensory difficulties" (2008, p. 10).

Practitioners of rehabilitation psychology must be cognizant of the effects of their choice of terms to describe test performance. Phrases such as "moderately impaired" and "below expectation" are common parlance in rehabilitation, but these terms imply somewhat different ranges ("below expectation" could apply to a wider range of scores than "moderately impaired"), and both of these "impairment" schemes suggest different standards of comparison for current performance than do "normative" descriptors such as "low average" or "superior (Caplan, 1995)." Mixing the various terminological typologies, common in clinical settings (Guilmette, Hagan, & Giuliano, 2008), can cause confusion. For example, a "low average" reading score could be viewed as "within expectation" for a high school dropout but "below expectation" or "severely impaired" for an individual with a graduate degree in English. The finding by Guilmette et al. of the greatest variability in use of "impairment" (vs. "normative") descriptors is especially relevant in rehabilitation, given the fact that many clients are there precisely because of conditions that compromise cognitive function and that will produce low test scores.

Sexual Functioning

Assessment of sexual functioning in rehabilitation populations presupposes familiarity with a medical literature that is alien to most other psychological specialties, as each major disabling condition is accompanied by its own set of facts and implications for sexual responsiveness and performance. However, this database is more critical for the intervention phase during which the psychologist would likely be discussing practical strategies and tactics for resumption of sexual expression as well as issues such as fertility and pregnancy. The content and process of assessment in this domain will at least partially resemble those used with other patient groups, as the rehabilitation psychologist seeks through interview to identify the sexual interests and usual practices of the particular individual and his or her partner. Knowledge of realistic options available to those with various types of disabilities is still important in this phase, as the psychologist must determine the patient's level of understanding of his or her condition as well as the likely effects on sexual activities. For example, as spinal cord injuries at different neurological levels carry different prognoses for erectile function, it is important that the psychologist understand and be able to convey clearly the difference between "psychogenic" and "reflex" erections and consequences for fertility of various injury levels.

Given the sensitivity of the topic, questions about sexuality rarely arise during initial sessions and, in fact, may not come up at all. Some patients will feel more comfortable asking for this information from their physicians. The topic may surface during the more intimate aspects of nursing care or therapy (e.g., an occupational therapist working with a patient on bathing techniques), and psychologists should be prepared to assist other staff members in dealing calmly and competently with the patient's questions and concerns. Nonetheless, it often falls to the psychologist to "give permission" for discussion of sex, incorporating the subject as naturally as possible into routine interview and/or educational counseling sessions, perhaps characterizing it as another "activity of daily living" that may be affected by the patient's condition.

The journal *Sexuality and Disability* is a useful resource, and condition-specific books (e.g., Griffith & Lemberg, 1993) or pamphlets (e.g., *Recovery After Stroke: Redefining Sexuality* from the National Stroke Association) can serve as jumping-off points for discussion.

Decision-Making Capacity

In light of the high frequency with which rehabilitation patients (often, but not exclusively, the elderly; American Bar Association and American Psychological Association, 2008; Moye, 1996; Moye, Amresto, & Karel, 2005) exhibit cognitive deficits, questions of various types of competence/capacity must be considered, and the rehabilitation psychologist has an important role to play in this effort. Although determination of competence is a legal action, not a psychological or medical one, the psychologist can speak to the issue of whether the individual has sufficient decision-making capacity to be declared competent for the particular purpose. (NB: Historically, the terms *competence* and *capacity* have been mistakenly used interchangeably, leading to considerable confusion.) As observed by Reid-Arndt et al. (2010, p. 88), it is the job of rehabilitation clinicians to "…supply the court with specific information about the nature, extent, and cause of incapacities and the prognosis (e.g., potential for recovery after TBI) as well as observations regarding perceived risk for poor decision-making in financial, health, personal care, and other relevant domains" (p. 88). Occasionally, "competence" can be lost and then regained (e.g., Marson et al., 2005), so serial assessment may be necessary.

It is important to keep in mind that "competence" is not a global condition but a specific one that requires a predicate—that is, one must be competent *for* something—for example, to manage finances, agree to (or refuse) treatment, drive, or sign a living will. Although neuropsychological tests and other evaluation protocols (e.g., Marson et al., 2000) may offer some basis for an opinion, direct questioning/discussion about the issue at hand may provide the most valid information. A useful approach involves exploring the patient's understanding of the clinical problem, treatment options, attendant risks and benefits, and likely outcome(s) as well as the reasoning underlying his or her choice. It is important to acknowledge that affected individuals can be competent to make decisions that appear to others to be unwise or risky. It may seem obvious, but in charged clinical situations, it can be tempting to conclude that a patient is not competent because he or she made an "inappropriate" decision (i.e., one with which the clinician or team disagrees). This temptation must be resisted or, at a minimum, its justification explored fully and the patient's reasoning determined.

The Uniform Guardianship and Protective Proceedings Act (2009) provides a useful general definition, characterizing an incapacitated person as one who "... is unable to receive and evaluate information or make or communicate decisions to such an extent that the individual lacks the ability to meet essential requirements for physical health, safety or self care, even with appropriate technological assistance." However, as definitions of "capacity" vary across states, the rehabilitation psychologist must be familiar with his or her home state guidelines. Some may require competence with respect to *outcome* (a reasonable decision), whereas others may hold to a lesser standard of competent *process* (i.e., informed decision).

Performance on neuropsychological tests may be so impaired as to support a position that the individual lacks requisite capacity. However, it is generally preferable to buttress this view with behavioral observations and evaluations of functional abilities as well as specific querying to elucidate the reasoning underlying the patient's position, understanding of likely consequences, and so forth. As many available tests do not necessarily carry ecological validity for this purpose, measures such as the Financial Capacity Instrument (Marson et al., 2000) and Independent Living Scales (Loeb, 2003) should be considered. In addition, some will find the MacArthur Scales (which use a structured interview format) helpful in probing the patient's understanding (Schaefer, 2010).

Of particular interest and relevance here is the guideline developed under the auspices of the Department of Veterans Affairs (1997) for evaluation of competency in the elderly. The guideline outlines a five-step process, the assessment portion of which entails a clinical interview; performance-based testing of cognition, functional abilities, and decision making; and assessment of mental health. Practitioners are advised to consider potential confounds such as psychomotor retardation, sensory impairments, and cultural factors. Clearly, the guideline embodies the broad biopsychosocial perspective characteristic of rehabilitation psychology.

Pain Assessment

It is the atypical rehabilitation patient that is completely pain free, although causes and courses can be quite varied (M. Robinson & O'Brien, 2010). Whatever the etiology, pain can certainly hinder the best rehabilitation efforts. Pain in the elderly has been especially underdiagnosed (Yonan & Wegener, 2003), particularly among those who may have difficulty communicating their discomfort because of cognitive impairment. In such instances, the rehabilitation psychologist may need to look to chart notes and behavioral observations (e.g., facial grimacing, groaning, squirming) to determine whether problematic pain exists (Hill-Briggs, Kirk, & Wegener, 2005).

Often, pain is adequately relieved through pharmacologic means, but persistent, disabling pain may require multipronged intervention. Contemporary approaches to the treatment of persons with a primary diagnosis of chronic pain embody the biopsychosocial model par excellence. In such instances, the information gleaned through psychological and behavioral assessment is essential in understanding the determinants of pain and how best to intervene.

There is no laboratory test for pain, as it is a subjective phenomenon; hence, pain assessment occurs primarily through patient self-report, although confirmation (or refutation) by informed collaterals and other observers such as therapists and nurses can be most informative. The challenges are nonetheless enormous, as patient–proxy agreement is often low (McPherson & Addington-Hall, 2003), and reported pain level may not always affect behavior; also, there are important individual differences in pain tolerance.

Although one may begin by administering such measures as the McGill Pain Questionnaire (Melzack, 2005) or visual analog or numerical rating scales (Jensen & Karoly, 2001) to identify the nature, location, and intensity of pain, instruments such as the West Haven-Yale Multidimensional

Pain Inventory (Kerns, Turk, & Rudy, 1985) and Survey of Pain Attitudes (Jensen & Karoly, 2007) will yield a broader picture of such factors as the patient's experience of pain, its impact on daily life activities, responses of significant others to pain behavior, views of treatment options, and expectations about possibility of improvement. Observation of variations in pain experience and behavior as a function of setting can be of great value in identifying important environmental influences (e.g., worsening of pain behavior in the presence of an overly solicitous spouse).

Doleys (2000) proposed that assessment of pain should consider that psychological/behavioral factors may play one or more of three roles in the development and "life" of chronic pain: mediating, modulating, or maintaining—that is, whether the factor in question intervenes between the precipitating event and appearance of pain; serves to attenuate or exacerbate pain when it is present; or contributes to the maintenance of chronic pain. Interested readers are referred to Doleys and Doherty (2000) and Jensen and Karoly (2001) for more detailed treatments of specific psychological instruments for measurement of pain.

Substance Use or Abuse Identification and Assessment

A regrettable number of individuals earn their status as "rehabilitation patient" with the help of intoxicating or otherwise mind-altering substances. In particular, for those with spinal cord injuries or traumatic brain injuries (some with both), alcohol and/or drugs will frequently have played an etiologic role (Bombardier & Turner, 2010). Furthermore, many conditions and/or treatments mandate minimization or avoidance of substance use after discharge; for instance, alcohol may compromise—or potentiate—the effects of certain medications, causing avoidable complications. In addition, there is evidence that those with substance misuse tendencies preinjury are at greater risk for both slower progress in rehabilitation and for postinjury misuse as well (Bombardier, Rimmele, & Zintel, 2002; Bombardier, Stroud, Esselman, & Rimmele, 2004). Therefore, a good substance use history is an important part of an initial rehabilitation psychology assessment.

Given the sensitivity of the subject and the potential for unpleasant consequences, it might seem reasonable to doubt whether patients would acknowledge what in retrospect is dangerous, irresponsible, or illegal behavior. However, studies (e.g., Cooney, Zweben, & Fleming, 1995) suggest that adequate techniques will elicit honest responses even from problem drinkers. Patients may well wonder if their insurance coverage is at risk if they admit to such behavior. As relevant laws vary by state, it is incumbent upon the psychologist to become familiar with local regulations (see Rivara, Tollefson, Tesh, & Gentilello, 2000, for discussion of this potentially thorny issue). Whatever the circumstances, a logical first step is chart review to determine whether alcohol or drugs were contributing factors at onset. Blood test results may be available as well as information about the patient's appearance and behavior at the time of injury and any prior discussion of substance use. The next step would be direct inquiry during the initial interview about use of alcohol and/or drugs just prior to onset as well as customary use, with self-report to be confirmed or refuted by discussion with close relatives or friends.

Although Rohe et al. (2002) reported considerable improvement during the preceding 15 years in the assessment of chemical health in rehabilitation settings, a recent survey (Cardoso, Pruett, Chan, & Tansey, 2006) found that many rehabilitation psychologists feel ill-equipped to deal with this topic. However, Bombardier and Turner (2010) argued that problems with substance abuse among rehabilitation populations are sufficiently similar to those in other psychological disorders that even persons without rehabilitation-specific training can learn to offer effective services.

Several short screening measures exist, although much of the information contained in these instruments can be obtained through interview (see Table 14.4 in Bombardier & Turner, 2010). For example, the CAGE questionnaire (Ewing, 1984) consists of four questions that could easily be incorporated into the initial or subsequent discussion. The Alcohol Use Disorders Identification Test (Allen, Litten, Fertig, & Babor, 1997) contains 10 items concerning consumption problems associated with alcohol use and symptoms of dependence. Fewer instruments exist to evaluate drug use, but the Alcohol, Smoking, and Substance Involvement Screening Test (ASSIST; WHO ASSIST Working Group, 2002) offers a comprehensive assessment.

Social and Behavioral Functioning

Successful rehabilitation hinges on cooperation between and among all involved—patient, family, and treatment team members. This alliance can be sabotaged by "problem behaviors" exhibited by patients that may antagonize staff, perhaps even causing them to retreat from involvement and unwittingly provide less than their best therapeutic efforts. Poor motivation, easy irritability, sexually provocative comments or actions, and denial are just a few of the behaviors that can earn one the tag of "problem patient." The rehabilitation psychologist who is an active member of the team—visible on the nursing unit and in the therapy gym, participating in patient rounds and staff conferences, asking about patient progress—will be made aware of problem situations via direct observation and "curbside consults" requested by frustrated therapists.

One important role the psychologist can play is that of "reframer," that is, suggesting alternative ways of understanding certain behaviors, when justified. This may amount to no more than using different terminology (Caplan & Shechter, 1993), positing, for example, that an "unmotivated" patient appears so because of depression, fatigue, or other factors. A stroke patient may seem "depressed" because of aprosodic speech despite normal mood. Encouraging staff to entertain these "rival hypotheses" about patient behavior is another unique contribution of the rehabilitation psychologist.

Conclusion

The importance to rehabilitation psychology of competence in assessment is underscored by the fact that in the ABRP board certification process, every skill related to assessment is deemed to be an "essential competency," the only such category. Of course, depending on the practitioner's particular setting, some of the competencies discussed in this chapter will be more or less important on a day-to-day basis. However, there is a long-standing consensus that the skilled advanced-level rehabilitation psychologist should be equipped to conduct assessments in all of these areas, should any presenting patient require this service. The preceding discussion serves to elucidate the multiple aspects, targets, and outcomes of the assessment process in rehabilitation psychology.

SEVEN

Consultation

This chapter provides an overview of the process of consultation as practiced by the rehabilitation psychologist. The word *consultation* takes on various meanings depending on the context and discipline. Consultation in psychology often has a different connotation than it does in the business world. Psychologists (and physicians) generally think of consultation in terms of clinical involvement, a three-party matrix that connects patient, therapist, and expert consultant. This triangular relationship is present in all consultation activities, as is the notion that services will typically be provided to the client/patient directly primarily by the treating professional and largely indirectly by the consultant (Frew, 2010).

Although this definition is often applicable, rehabilitation consultation work will occasionally be more extensive and inclusive. The rehabilitation psychologist consultant may be advising a much larger treatment matrix—for instance, several individuals from differing professions or a multidisciplinary rehabilitation team. Consultation may even include organizational and/or administrative persons representing treatment facilities or fundraising/advocacy organizations. Meeting the needs of the patient is always paramount, but to do so, it is frequently necessary simultaneously to address the needs of staff and team members (Diller, 1990).

One caveat: Certain circumstances may dictate that a rehabilitation psychology "consultant" act more like a member of the permanent team than an outside expert—for example, in a rural area where the team might have no regular psychological services or when the team psychologist is on vacation. In such instances, the consultant may be asked (required?) to provide direct services such as assessment or counseling.

The Team

The team approach to treatment has been a basic feature of rehabilitation for decades. Although psychologists historically were considered "core" members of that team (Butt & Caplan, 2010, p. 451), in some settings economic factors now dictate a consultative role for the psychologist. Several models of team involvement are found in the literature, and multiple models may exist even within a single treatment facility. For instance, an institution's burn unit team might have a different makeup than their spinal cord injury treatment team. Teams generally consist of persons working in the same facility, but other organizations may supply professionals from "missing" disciplines in response to a unique clinical situation.

Treatment Models

Butt and Caplan (2010) describe the several models of teams as differing largely in the distinctiveness of the roles of the providers and the treatment goals toward which they are working with the patient: *multidisciplinary*—there is collaboration between different disciplines, each of which may be working in a different role and having different patient goals; *interdisciplinary*—the roles and functions of the collaborating clinicians overlap somewhat; *transdisciplinary*—the various disciplines have significant overlap in the roles and the patient goals that they are working toward. Each model will present unique and special concerns and challenges for the rehabilitation psychologist consultant.

Because every treatment model has its own inherent strengths and weaknesses, the consultant should be conversant with the various models, as well as equipped to help develop "one off" models for especially complicated cases. Models are often like rules, that is, useful to set guidelines and get started, but not immutable. Some systems become so entrenched in their particular invented, adopted, and/or stylized model that deviance from it is not well received. The adroit consultant recognizes and corrects such behavior so as not to inhibit the patient's progress.

The Consultant

The work of the consultant in rehabilitation psychology represents a very broad spectrum of skills, factual information, and administrative savvy. The term *consultant* literally means "calling together the senate" (*consultare senatorum*). This analogy is particularly applicable to rehabilitation psychology in that "team" work is the assembling of a collaborative interaction of professionals from various disciplines to intervene on behalf of a client.

Consultation demands a spectrum of knowledge that is extremely broad, including, but not limited to, concepts and processes from social work, physical therapy, legal services, religious/spiritual concerns, nursing, many specialties within medicine, psychological specialties other than rehabilitation (e.g., neuropsychology, health psychology, school psychology), occupational therapy, and other adjunctive therapies. Although rehabilitation psychologists need not have detailed knowledge of other disciplines, they must be sufficiently acquainted with what these specialties offer and how and when to refer to and collaborate with them. Team meetings, case conferences, and grand rounds offer excellent opportunities to both learn the unique offerings of other disciplines and discover ways to include them for the patient's benefit.

The following are reasonable expectations of the consulting rehabilitation psychologist:

1. Respond in a timely fashion, usually within 24 hours, with at least a preliminary report
2. Know and follow ethical guidelines including those pertaining to releases of information, confidentiality, professional decorum, boundaries, etc.
3. Know the relevant federal, state, and other applicable laws
4. Be able to write a concise, yet informative and useful, final report
5. Know the limits of one's ability
6. Be aware of professionals who can assist beyond the consultant's own competencies.

The rehabilitation psychologist is likely to be called upon to deal with a wide spectrum of disabilities, diseases, illness conditions, and emotional/personality issues. The work of the consultant may not end when the primary referral question has been addressed. To address the referral question and its ramifications initially, adequately, and completely, exploration into educational, family, work history, social functioning, and even legal issues frequently becomes necessary, and this process may bring to light other matters (perhaps related to the original problem but perhaps not) that require intervention. Collateral information is often indispensable.

Novack, Sherer, and Penna (2010) write regarding history taking per se, but their observation applies to consultation situations as well:

> Obtaining a thorough patient history can be a major contribution... supplementing the medical history by focusing on social history (particularly education and employment), substance abuse, daily activities, psychiatric background, coping capacity, and family history. It is important that family members and caregivers are interviewed in addition to the patient, as this contact allows confirmation (or refutation) of information given by the patient... (p. 166).

The consultant should know the availability of other professionals in the community, both psychologists and disciplines involved in the myriad needs of rehabilitation patients. Those working in smaller communities will be challenged to identify available diagnostic and treatment resources and frequently must familiarize themselves with more distant resources. In metropolitan areas, the consultant is more likely to have personal knowledge on which to act. The more common referral questions center around head injuries, spinal cord injuries, burns, strokes, dementias, vehicular injuries, and accidental fall injuries. However, as has been stated previously, the spectrum of diseases, illnesses, trauma, degenerative diseases, and medical conditions defies limitation. Consequently, the rehabilitation psychologist consultant should be informed about and connected with as many resources as possible.

Although there are many and varied disability classifications, competencies are addressed within the framework of expected services of the consulting rehabilitation psychologist; therefore, all areas, regardless of diagnostic or disability classification, require the following capabilities:

1. Thorough review of the referral question to be certain of what is being asked; obtaining clarification, as needed
2. Developing rapport with the patient and family
3. Determining the method of assessment
4. Identifying the primary (and possible secondary) problem(s)
5. Considering differential diagnosis, preferably arriving at a working diagnosis
6. If indicated and requested, determining a plan of intervention/treatment

7. Conceptualizing/completing a report (often preceded by a preliminary report)

In a certain sense, all consultation could be classified under Caplan's schema for "mental health" because it offers a workable framework for consultation in most situations. The rehabilitation psychologist, while perhaps emphasizing mental health or other psychological matters, must operate within a much broader framework. Caplan (1995, pp. 7–21) lists four types of mental health, and the framework is adaptable for any kind of consultation:

1. Client centered
2. Program centered
3. Consultee personal/skill concerns
4. Consultee administrative matters

In terms of importance, all are equivalent. However, in rehabilitation psychology *consultation,* clarifying the referral question is initially primary, for example, making certain of the *primary question* and what it is that the referring source *wants* and *needs from the consultant that cannot be obtained elsewhere.* Once that is established, a clear route for discovery and implementation may be developed and initiated.

Fostering effective communication among the referring source, team members, consultant, organization (hospital or rehabilitation setting), patient, other disciplines outside the immediate rehabilitation team, and patient's family is a fundamental responsibility of the rehabilitation psychologist consultant. When team members are engaged in "committee-type" problem solving, complications may emerge not only from communication difficulties but also from varying conceptualizations of the basic problem. Having a team leader (often the psychologist) is key to clarifying and implementing the ultimate team consensus.

Potential Concerns

Potential problems arise at many levels. The referral question may have been inadequately framed and the initial assessment therefore of little value. The assessment process may be culpable if the guidelines are insufficiently precise and/or if a faulty systemic approach is utilized. The individual responsible for the initial assessment may not have had the time, resources, training, or experience to gather adequate information to clarify the problem, its etiology, and other factors necessary to clearly formulate the referral question, let alone offer information beneficial to the consultant. Nonetheless, the consultant psychologist will be expected to proceed regardless of the adequacy (or lack thereof) of the initial evaluation. Not all referral sources will have the breadth and depth of information that would be helpful to the consultant. Often organizational structures and job descriptions prevent initial providers from doing all they would like or know how to do.

Further, rehabilitation is frequently a slow process; gains are made in "baby steps," each requiring careful planning, often taking more than the expected time, and demanding more expertise than might be imagined from persons not intimately acquainted with the rehabilitation process.

Following are some of the basic areas considered by the American Board of Rehabilitation Psychology (ABRP) to be common, but not exclusive or exhaustive, areas that the rehabilitation psychologist consultant should be prepared to encounter.

Behavioral Functioning

Consulting regarding behavioral functioning is extremely broad, encompassing any and all behaviors that may be beneficial or compromising for successful rehabilitation. We discuss here just a few of the major behavior challenges that may arise. The consultant is reasonably expected to discover the hurdles of emotional (i.e., mental health/illness) and physical problem areas, as well as to aid in effective planning and treatment.

Poor compliance with—or avoidance of—treatment is common. However, although compliance/noncompliance is frequently discussed in medical management, it is rarely mentioned in rehabilitation literature as a distinct issue in spite of the fact that noncompliance is prevalent and frequently the most significant hindrance to rehabilitation. The etiology of noncompliance may be obvious (e.g., excessive fatigue, pain) or require considerable delving to detect. It is important to differentiate "noncompliance" or "poor motivation" or "obstinance" from avoidance behavior triggered by such factors as depression, pain, cognitive dysfunction (especially impaired awareness), medication/drugs, personnel conflicts, and misunderstandings, including marital, domestic, and environmental dysfunction. The skilled rehabilitation psychology consultant will consider "alternative vocabularies" in explaining difficult patient behavior (Caplan & Shechter, 1993), a tactic that may lead to deeper understanding of root causes and, hence, more effective intervention.

Poor compliance is not necessarily of patient origin; it may derive from an uninspiring and/or poorly functioning rehabilitation team, personality conflicts with and within staff, suboptimal environmental conditions such as hospital wards, patient–family dysfunction, and numerous other factors. What appears to be noncompliance may be a consequence of a program that is understaffed, thus not allowing sufficient one-on-one time for patients who do not do well in group settings. Mobilizing the patient's family as copartners in their family member's care can promote a patient's willingness to be compliant with treatment. As consultant, "The rehabilitation psychologist can assist in managing the sometimes fractious relations that develop between staff and patient and/or his or her family, fostering a better communication and understanding of the other 'team members" stresses, motivations, concerns, and behavior" (Caplan & Reidy, 1996, p. 21).

A competent consultant recognizes that what appears to be avoidance may be a reaction to ambiguity, misunderstandings, or mixed, opposing, or incompatible messages from team members to the patient. Care must be taken to foster consistency and focus upon a single, clearly understood, and uniformly implemented treatment plan. This is a major function of team meetings and case conferences, and a key function of the team leader is to assist in establishing and maintaining the consistent approach of the team as a whole. However, the fresh eyes of a consultant can sometimes detect factors overlooked by the team.

A patient's inability or unwillingness to adhere to schedules can become disruptive and sabotage the best treatment plan. Patients with head injuries or strokes, for example, may have a distorted sense of time, be unable to understand or keep schedules, and may even suffer nocturnal/diurnal reversals, giving rise to sleep disorders that can prevent adherence to a schedule. Sleep disorders may go unrecognized, particularly in a hospital setting where sedatives are apt to be administered routinely, thus masking and/or producing sleep problems. Sleep deprivation can be most disruptive causing inadequate rest, REM state disturbances, and eating and other bodily function disturbances; this is especially pertinent for older adults (Stepanski, Rybarczyk, Lopez, & Stevens, 2003) . Sleep disorders may be assessed by various means including "sleep clinics," "sleep laboratories," and the *Sleep Disorders Inventory for Students* (Luginbuehl, 2008).

Consultation requests are frequently triggered by aggressive behavior, a belligerent attitude, insulting remarks, sexual provocation, and a confrontational stance from the patient, often—but by no means exclusively—from survivors of traumatic brain injury for whom disinhibition is a common problem. In such instances, the consultant must attempt to determine the root cause of this disruptive behavior—for example, brain injury, masked depression, or lifelong obstreperousness. It must be remembered that "...anger, aggression (turned inwardly and resulting in feeling of guilt and shame, or turned outwardly to trigger feelings of other-blame and need for revenge) are common responses to disability adaptation" (Hanoch & Siller, 2004, p. 36). A competent and seasoned staff is expected to deal with aggressive and even insulting behavior objectively, without personalizing the affront and without prejudice.

Insulting and aggressive behavior can arise from sources other than the patient—for example, from family members who are in grief, angered over the many factors producing and arising from disability, and even from staff who may overidentify and displace their feelings onto others. The rehabilitation psychologist consultant—as one who is not enmeshed in the day-to-day interpersonal interactions and clashes on the unit—may offer a more objective perspective on underlying causes of behavioral problems.

Interpersonal relationships among family members may also be a source of behavioral complications requiring input from a psychology consultant. Traumatic incidents may arouse latent problems, causing re-emergence of dormant dysfunctional family interactions and causing old hurts to resurface. Even healthy family functioning can be disrupted by trauma-induced role shifts or reversals affecting both patients and family members, with the latter possibly fearing the difficulties of caregiving after their loved one's discharge.

Cultural and Language Concerns

Cultural factors must be taken into account when appraising the "appropriateness" of behavior. Language that is common in one cultural setting may be unacceptable in another. A similar contingency applies to actions and behaviors that may appear rude or even aggressive in one locale but not another. Some assert that culture helps define what individuals believe, perceive, value, and know even as early as age 5 (Lynch & Hanson, 2004). Understanding the patient's background requires more than is typically included in a medical or psychological history but should be considered by the skilled rehabilitation consultant.

In a multiethnic population, language becomes a significant consideration. Patients and families whose first language is not that of the dominant culture, and who may have only a marginal knowledge of the same, present special challenges. Even when everyone is speaking the same language, this does not mean they are communicating clearly and unambiguously. Unless the parties share an understanding of culturally shaped meanings for words or phrases—particularly idioms and regional expressions—conversational havoc may result, leading to unintended consequences. "Repetition is our friend" serves as a reminder of the importance of being "redundant" in the service of ensuring a common understanding. Asking the other party to repeat what they have heard allows the consultant to detect and correct faulty grasp of facts, further fostering accurate communication.

Although an individual rehabilitation psychology consultant cannot be expected to be familiar with every culture and cultural nuance that may be encountered, one should strive toward the practice of "culturally informed" psychology. Chapter 3 on individual and cultural diversity in this volume cites several references that can provide a good starting point from which to work.

Cognitive Functioning

Although the subject of a particular consultation request may not be cognitive function per se, all patients must concentrate, think, understand instructions, work through problems, and so forth. Hence, the consultant almost invariably assesses cognition, even if incidentally or informally. The consultant must carefully analyze sources and etiology of "cognitive deficits" before offering recommendations for remediation. Even conditions that are primarily physical in nature may also involve concomitant traumatic brain injury, chemical or drug-induced difficulties, residua from high fevers or anesthesia, and other factors secondary to the primary problem; all of these can result in impaired cognition.

Common situations in which the consultation is related to cognition include: (a) collaborating with occupational and speech therapists in deriving a coherent understanding of a patient's cognitive functioning (these other disciplines employ their own means of assessing cognition, but they tend not to evaluate memory or executive functioning, both of which have significant implications for rehabilitation); (b) assisting physical and occupational therapists in understanding how a patient's cognitive limitations affect such matters as their capacity to understand directions or remember how to perform therapeutic activities from one session to another; (c) detecting unusual neuropsychological presentations that might have been overlooked by others; (d) identifying neuropsychological phenomena that have been misinterpreted (e.g., a patient whose speech is aprosodic may incorrectly be assumed to be apathetic or depressed); and (e) helping staff to select and implement interventions that consider the patient's cognitive level.

A psychology consultant can also aid the team by correcting certain "common sense" notions that are, in fact, not supported by psychological research. Consider the following example that relates to an aspect of cognition. It is an old saw in rehabilitation that patients should be given as many choices as feasible, because their disability may have taken away numerous freedoms and options they previously enjoyed. This well-meaning and seemingly benign position fails to take account of the phenomenon of "decisional fatigue." Research by Baumeister and his colleagues (e.g., Vohs et al., 2008) has found that as people are required to make a series of decisions, a sort of cognitive fatigue sets in, and their choices become more automatic and less thoughtful. They cite findings that "…suggest that choice, to the extent that it requires greater decision making among options, can become burdensome and ultimately counterproductive" (p. 884).

Vocational and Educational Issues

Depending primarily on the age of the client, educational or vocational rehabilitation concerns may prompt requests for input from a rehabilitation psychology consultant. Although historically there was a strong link between rehabilitation psychology and vocational rehabilitation, this competency currently receives rather less attention in doctoral training programs than those designated as "clinical" areas. Nonetheless, vocational rehabilitation remains an important part of the rehabilitation psychologist's role in many cases, as educational or vocational restoration (encompassing all kinds of productive activity) is a major goal for many rehabilitation participants.

It is not possible to overemphasize the place of education in rehabilitation. The "learning role" is essential in every phase of treatment involving new skill learning, acquisition of new attitudes and values that take the disabling condition into account, new approaches to physical activity, and much more.

Testing for aptitude, interest, and adaptability for various occupations or to identify helpful accommodations for return to school may take place during rehabilitation (more likely on an outpatient basis). The rehabilitation psychology consultant can then serve as an intermediary with the school or potential employer to convey the assessment results and their implications as well as suggestions for implementation that may include recommendations for accommodations.

The rehabilitation psychology consultant should be conversant with resources for both training and vocational opportunities such as the *Occupational Handbook*, published by the U.S. Department of Labor (every 2 years), an essential tool that is now online (http://www.bls.gov/oco/). The U.S. Department of Labor offers many resources for educational/vocational planning. Parents of children with traumatic brain injury who are returning to school may benefit from educational/consultation programs such as BrainSTARS (Dise-Lewis, Lewis, & Reichardt, 2009). Schools and employers may require reminders about their obligations to provide reasonable accommodations under the Americans With Disabilities Act. Rehabilitation psychology consultants can also direct clients to potential funding resources, particularly for those physically challenged, from both the state and federal government.

Dealing With Pain

Many conditions encountered in rehabilitation psychology practice are accompanied by pain; indeed, some individuals enter rehabilitation specifically for treatment of chronic pain (M. Robinson & O'Brien, 2010). It is important for the consultant to recognize the many levels and causes for pain; often, the etiology is multifactorial. Further, because there is no accepted objective measurement of pain, it remains a subjective evaluation by the patient. It is this subjective character that treating staff frequently find most frustrating (even annoying), especially when pain interferes with participation in therapy. The rehabilitation psychology consultant provides a tremendous service to patients and staff alike by reinforcing the lessons of Fordyce's (1976) work on behavioral treatment of chronic pain—namely, an approach that seeks to identify factors that elicit and perpetuate pain behavior and employs behavioral targets and time-dependent (not pain-dependent) administration of medication.

Neuropathic pain, which is chronic disabling pain, is the most challenging and presents the greatest hindrances for rehabilitation. Pain syndromes must not be lumped together but carefully analyzed in the light of physiology, medications, lifestyle, psychological status, and implications for educational, vocational, and life-skills remediation. There are multiple sequelae to pain, most of which disrupt both lifestyle and rehabilitation efforts. The most common concerns revolve around dependency (learned disability), drug misuse and abuse (prescription, over the counter, legal, and illegal), and depression.

Although there is usually a distinct differentiation between emotional pain and physical pain, the two tend to be intertwined. Frequently the consulting rehabilitation psychologist will be of great value in pain management due to his or her behavioral expertise and insight into the psychodynamics of pain as well as the ability to organize a team and utilize a broad background of multidisciplinary knowledge to orchestrate an intervention.

Pain and discomfort become daily companions of many rehabilitation clients. Adjusting to new levels of pain tolerance, dealing with the side effects and complications of pain medications, avoiding addiction to narcotics, and accommodating to a lifestyle that requires "pushing through" pain are a few of the challenges related to pain and the rehabilitation patient. The competent psychologist, in tandem with the patient's physician, can often ameliorate some of the pain and almost always assist in the psychological management of pain and its sequelae. The consultant must also be aware of the many discomforts that may not be currently painful but can become so (e.g., infections, indwelling catheters, wheelchairs, assistive devices, orthotics).

Laws and Advocacy

The reader is referred to a more thorough discussion of regulations and laws found in Chapter 2 (on ethical and legal issues) of this volume. The consultant will, at a minimum, be aware of the basic legal requirements for rehabilitation. Laws, rules, and regulations change; therefore, diligence is required to keep abreast of the rights and limitations of both the professional and the patient. A further and important consideration in all consultation is the aspect of being an effective advocate working for consumer protection. Becoming a contributor, advisor, or committee member or having other involvement in organizations that advocate for the challenged and/or disadvantaged in our society is considered by many to be an ethical responsibility of professionals in psychology.

Some rehabilitation psychologists may be called upon to provide a life-planning report, which will include everything from living accommodations to financial requirements. Vocational considerations become particularly important—whether the patient will be able to return to a previous occupation (with or without accommodation), need to move to an alternative line of work utilizing previously learned skills, learn an entirely new occupation with new skills, or be able to be gainfully employed in any occupation.

Rehabilitation psychologists are often consulted to provide input regarding disability as it relates to accommodations in the workplace and/or provision of benefits under disability policies such as Social Security Disability (Cox & Goldberg, 2010). Such consultation requires not only the clinical expertise to assess a patient's status but also substantial knowledge of the laws, rules, and regulations pertaining to determination of disability.

Personality/Emotional Status

Because trauma and resultant disability typically cause strong emotional reactions and may even affect long-standing personality traits (albeit not necessarily so; see Kurtz, Putnam, & Stone, 1998), the rehabilitation consultant can assume that these factors will need careful diagnostic attention. The astute clinician will strive to distinguish carefully between the two, because emotional states tend to be transient and more susceptible to modification. As with other phenomena, individual differences in cultural background, religious beliefs, gender, and premorbid personality may shape differing interpretations of disability and rehabilitation generally and one's own in particular, giving rise to differing emotional conclusions and states.

The consultant should endeavor to gain some insight into the patient's premorbid personality, especially with respect to matters such as stress tolerance, optimism/pessimism, and coping style, as this information will inform management recommendations made to the treating team. Although one might assume that severe trauma would routinely produce alterations in personality, there is evidence that lifelong characteristics may endure even after traumatic brain injury (Kurtz, Putnam, & Stone, 1998); in some cases, there may be exacerbation of pretrauma traits, such that an intermittently irascible individual becomes chronically irritable. Interviews with family members, friends, or colleagues will likely be useful in this effort.

The rehabilitation psychology consultant may be confronted with requests to assist in management of many varieties of emotional responses to new-onset disability, depression and anxiety almost certainly being the most common. Review of chart notes can illuminate the nature of the problem—for example, is the referral source's concern about "depression" based on patient statements demonstrating dejection and despondency, behaviors such as poor cooperation in therapy, or signs such as sleep disruption or poor appetite? This information will help the consultant determine whether to focus on emotional state or behaviors.

Psychological terminology having become commonplace in ordinary discourse, there is a risk that "psychological" or "behavioral" terms may be misused by staff, and the consultant can serve a valuable function by reinterpreting (and correcting) these errors (Caplan & Shechter, 1993). For example, suicidal thoughts are often perceived by staff in statements such as "I don't know how I can live this way." For some, this is, indeed, equivalent to "I wish I had died in the accident," but for many it is a literal expression of ignorance—they truly do not understand what life after rehabilitation could consist of. This provides the consultant (or any staff member) an opportunity to educate them in general terms about rehabilitation therapies as learning experiences preparing them for postdischarge life. The rehabilitation psychologist consultant can "reframe" such ideation as a "normal response to an abnormal situation/event," potentially enlightening the patient, calming the family, *and* increasing the psychological sophistication of the staff.

Likewise, help may be requested in managing a patient's (or relatives') anxiety. Some anxieties encountered in rehabilitation patients may be exacerbations of previously subclinical entities that have been exaggerated by trauma, but many more derive from the complicated concerns of regaining and maintaining health, inconveniences of daily living (for instance, inaccessibility of the home), and ambiguities related to future employment, education, and social and interpersonal relationships. Here again, the patient's state can be characterized as a "knowledge deficit" that is susceptible to education and reassurance that most of the patient's questions and concerns can be addressed in some fashion.

Bodily disfigurement from burns, amputations, surgeries, and other illnesses or injuries can produce discernible emotional disturbances. It is important to consider whether the disability was traumatically induced (as in an automobile accident or chemical explosion) or due to something such as surgical removal of a limb, as in diabetic complications; among other distinctions, the latter can be anticipated but not the former, so each presents a different scenario in terms of emotional dynamics. The issue of personal responsibility for the disabling condition may be paramount and may interact with religious/spiritual beliefs. If a devout individual is injured by someone else's hand, a distressing feeling of "divine betrayal" may take hold, producing withdrawal and depression; alternatively, the event may be seen as a "test" of one's beliefs, fostering motivation for rehabilitation.

Substance Use/Abuse

The topic of substance use and misuse is most relevant to all phases of the rehabilitation process. Many disability-causing events were triggered by alcohol or drug use. Continuing indulgence (abetted by outside accomplices) during rehabilitation can complicate or sabotage progress; this situation—troublesome and frustrating for staff—often prompts introduction of a psychology consultant. In certain conditions (e.g., brain injury), use of alcohol and/or recreational drugs is strongly contraindicated because of potentially dangerous interactions as well as the possibility of further injury due to alcohol- or drug-fueled disinhibited behavior. Bombardier and Turner (2010) discuss models for assessment and evaluation for substance abuse as well as intervention using the technique of motivational interviewing. The consultant can play an important part in minimizing substance misuse by educating patients and families, guiding them to outpatient treatment programs, and helping to reduce logistical barriers (Corrigan, Bogner, Lamb-Hart, Heinemann, & Moore, 2005). Bombardier and Turner (2010) note that, although many psychologists believe that working in the area of substance misuse demands special skills and knowledge, in fact, alcohol- and drug-related problems and behaviors frequently respond to the same kinds of interventions as do other psychological disorders.

Sexual Functioning

Most conditions encountered in rehabilitation have some implications for sexual expression and functioning. The rehabilitation psychologist called to consult on this topic must be conversant with a broad spectrum of knowledge about the impacts of disorders such as spinal cord injury, stroke, brain injury, and multiple sclerosis, to mention just a few. In these conditions, there are likely to be primary neurological effects on sexuality, whereas other conditions such as chronic pain or amputation are more likely to be accompanied by emotional responses concerning sexuality (although the affective realm is certainly not unaffected in those with neurological conditions).

Gender differences are to be expected. Distinctly female issues such as the onset of menarche/menstrual cycles, fertility, and concerns about pregnancy and delivery may be present (Nosek, 2010). Nosek (p. 373) reports that "Conventional social wisdom is that women with disabilities are often viewed as asexual, have no need for intimacy or sexual expression, and are incapable of being a sexual partner." This erroneous view—frequently shared by the patient and family—can be countered by the astute consultant. Males tend to have concerns regarding erectile ability, ejaculation, performance issues, and the viability of sperm.

Consults on matters of a sexual nature may be prompted by staff members holding attitudes about sex better suited to an earlier time. If patient inquiries about sex—even those that occur in situations where they might be expected (e.g., catheterizing a male with a spinal cord injury produces a reflex erection)—are discouraged because of staff discomfort, the patient thereby may infer that the topic is off limits and conclude that sexual activity may not be part of his or her future. A rehabilitation psychology consultant can counter this unfortunate misconception.

Given the sensitivity of the subject, staff members should be equipped to respond calmly if a given patient chooses to raise the topic with them, acknowledging their ignorance, if necessary, and soliciting outside input, perhaps from a consultant. It is desirable that all treating staff be capable of providing the first two levels of intervention in the well-known PLISSIT model (Annon, 1974) of sexual counseling—giving Permission, and providing Limited Information. The remaining levels (Specific Suggestions and Intensive Therapy) are perhaps best left to specialists.

Although somewhat tangential to the topic of sexuality, concerns related to parenting as a person with a disability are common, and the consultant can help patients think through the likely logistics of raising a child, given their own probable limitations. As identified by Sieh, Meijer, and Visser-Meily (2010), identification of depression in the stroke survivor can be a warning sign for stress and possible development of behavioral problems in (especially female) children.

Physical Functioning

The loss of bodily functioning is itself traumatic, although at each age, there are unique concerns. The child with a disability faces a lifetime of challenges, the adolescent may be deprived of participation in certain sports and social activities, the adult impaired for gainful employment, and the elderly individual experiencing an accelerated compromise of daily living skills. Psychology consultants need to adopt a developmental perspective to deal with concerns in this area.

Although physical limitations affect both male and female patients, the impairment(s) must be viewed within the context of their individual cultural, social, and age-related real and assumed needs. Physical limitations "that define disability affect women at higher rates as they age; increasing from 6% of women ages 18–44 to 40% of those age 65 or older" (Chevarley, 2006, p. 297). This may be related, at least in part, to limitations in resources such as income, access to insurance, and other such factors.

Physical limitations on mobility are of particular importance when the consultant is dealing with future employment possibilities and/or adjustment to current occupational demands. However, the implications of limitations on physical functioning are much more pervasive than just those relating to mobility. There may be increased susceptibility to diseases such as obesity and diabetes. Macular degeneration and other progressive visual disorders; age-related hearing loss; other degenerative sensory dysfunctions; age-related onset of hereditary and genetic disorders; cardiovascular, renal, and hepatic failure; and pulmonary and other organ dysfunctions become of even greater importance to those already physically compromised, as the body may have lost its ability to defend itself, resulting in a "domino effect" and downward spiral of health. Diet, exercise, and lifestyle—major concerns for all persons—become of vital importance to those for whom every physical problem magnifies the challenges already present. The "health psychology" component of the rehabilitation psychologist's knowledge base comes into play in addressing these matters.

Assistive Technology

The modern world of technology offers unprecedented advantages for those who are physically challenged. From bionic limbs to voice- and eye movement–controlled communication devices, persons who previously have endured handicaps can now take advantage of technological advances in amazing ways. For examples of this, the reader is referred to the very helpful overview of this area provided by Kirsch and Scherer (2010).

> Assistive Technology for Cognition and Behavior (ATCB) is a class of interventions that uses electronic devices to facilitate performance of functional tasks. Computerized devices and systems are central to ATCB applications because they provide a method for interacting with users automatically and for monitoring the user's behavior.... [L]ocal area wireless technologies have become increasingly common, both at home and in community settings. These networks can be used to design

interventions that interact with a user dynamically, rather than requiring that the user be dependent on off-line, static, device specific systems.... [G]eographically dispersed, wide area wireless networks are becoming available that permit continuous use of ATCB systems in locations far beyond the clinic.... (Furthermore), there have been significant advances in the miniaturization and power of environmental sensors that can automatically detect environmental changes so that interventions can be implemented and adjusted based on feedback about user's performance (Kirsch & Scherer, 2010, p. 273).

As well as the technologies themselves, the milieu, personal, and technology factors will need consideration. Significant education, monitoring, support, and technological information are needed by the user. Carefully matching the person and technology is critical to promote acceptance and actual use in daily life. Consultation in this area tends to be highly specialized involving clinical as well as technical knowledge.

Although most attention in the literature on rehabilitation is addressed to physical (i.e., movement) disabilities, advances in technology for cognitive problems and limitations of sight, hearing, and other senses should not be overlooked. For example, talking computers help the blind hear what they cannot see, and personal digital assistants can serve as external memory banks.

Assistive devices for mobility have also become technologically smart. Wheelchairs that climb steps are now available, as are limbs that move with mere thought as the directive, and cochlear implants that improve hearing for the hearing-impaired.

Cost can be a major consideration (and obstacle) when attempting to advise regarding assistive devices. The consultant rehabilitation psychologist may not be knowledgeable in this area and may need to enlist persons from the orthotic, orthopedic appliance, technology, and assistive devices world.

Finally, one might consult with respect to "assistive devices" that are nontechnical in nature—specifically, the possible value of assistance animals should not be overlooked (Sachs-Ericsson, Hansen, & Fitzgerald, 2002). Recent years have brought about an increase in the kinds of animals that are being trained and the disabilities for which they can be effective.

Although the consultant, in all likelihood, may not be an expert in the technology of assistive devices, maintaining a broad general acquaintance with the technologies available will be essential to the effective consultant.

On Being Agent

The importance and degree of professional responsibility of the rehabilitation psychologist consultant cannot be overstated and must not be underestimated by the consultant. The consultant rehabilitation psychologist becomes *agent*, usually *de facto*. Although not a legally binding conservatorship, it is a morally and professionally binding relationship. To accept the position of agent assumes the willingness to act at all times in the best interest of the person to whom one is agent, recognizing that often as agent the consultant is acting *instead of* the represented party due to the inability of that party to do so.

EIGHT

Consumer Protection

Rehabilitation psychologists are expected to be advocates for and protectors of the interests and well-being of consumers of rehabilitation psychology services. The concept of advocacy—albeit in a professional fashion—is integral in rehabilitation psychology, has been a long-standing aspect of the field, and has its roots in the very early days of the specialty.

The American Board of Rehabilitation Psychology expects that candidates for board certification in rehabilitation psychology demonstrate competency in consumer protection through (a) effective advocacy in laws related to and including the Americans With Disabilities Act (ADA), as well as (b) awareness and sensitivity to multicultural and diversity factors. The chapters in this text on legal/ethical matters (Chapter 2) and diversity (Chapter 3) present more specifics in those areas; the present chapter focuses on the concepts of consumer protection and advocacy in more general terms.

Consumer protection and advocacy can be demonstrated in a number of fashions: active participation in consumer groups; professional organizations on the local, state, and national levels; board certification and related academies; grassroots and/or legislative activity; provision of public education services; and more (Cox, 2010). Rehabilitation psychologists actively advocate for needed services and community supports for the patients they treat, focusing on the patient's ability to engage maximally in independent living and on increasing the patient's quality of life (Cox et al., 2010). Wright (1993, p. 65), in her remarks regarding the heritage of the American Psychological Association (APA) Division of Rehabilitation Psychology, reflected on how essential and fundamental the concepts of consumer protection and advocacy are in the specialty area; she essentially advocated for this to become "...a core requirement in the education and training of rehabilitation psychologists." She also indicated that despite differences of opinion among early rehabilitation psychologists regarding the definition of rehabilitation psychology, the field found consensus regarding characteristics of the specialty, of which this was one (Wright, 1959).

Artman and Daniels (2010), in a significant paper addressing the need for increased awareness and training of psychologists to work with persons with disabilities, note that although many other types of psychologists come into contact with persons with disabilities, the issue of disability is often directed to the specialty of rehabilitation psychology. They note that awareness and training in advocacy skills is essential in working with persons with disabilities. Many examples of perhaps basic, and often relatively easy-to-implement, actions can be undertaken to advocate for consumer/patient protections and rights. These include, among others, addressing accessibility issues in the facility in which one works; reviewing print and other materials for accessibility for individuals with low vision ; scheduling appointments that accommodate public transportation and patient fatigue levels throughout the day; sensitivity to the environmental issues such as lighting, temperature, space for wheelchairs, and so forth; and adaptation of testing materials (as addressed also in the assessment chapter (Chapter 6) of the present text). Psychologists need to become familiar with local resources that may facilitate the protection of rights of persons with disabilities. These may include legal services, information resources, and others. Examples are the Legal Aid Society, the Center for Independent Living, and state departments of vocational rehabilitation.

Advocating and Consumer Protection: Being Actively Involved

TOPICS OF ADVOCACY AND CONSUMER PROTECTION

There are several major areas in which advocacy and consumer protection are frequently called for in the field of rehabilitation psychology. Some of these follow and, as indicated earlier, the reader may find yet more information in the corresponding chapters (Chapters 2 and 3) of this book relating to legal issues and/or diversity.

Legal issues such as arise from the ADA, the Individuals With Disability Education Act (IDEA), and other outgrowths of our society's increased awareness of the needs and rights of persons with disabilities are constantly evolving. Interested readers might start with Bruyère and

O'Keefe's (1994) excellent text on the implications of the ADA. However, many changes have occurred since then, and rehabilitation psychologists must stay apprised of these; the website http://www.ada.gov is one place to access current information. Advocating for suitable accommodations in the workplace or educational setting is a common function of many rehabilitation psychologists. It is increasingly common for a rehabilitation psychologist to address specific needs and/or accommodations and to consult with schools, attorneys, and/or employers regarding these issues.

More often than not, the focus of the rehabilitation psychologist, then, is directly on the patient–employment or patient–environment interaction, at the individual level. However, effecting change through groups and professional areas of study/investigation is also a critical element of the advocacy agenda. Lollar (2008) describes a pivotal role that rehabilitation psychology as a field can bring to society, particularly as it interacts with public health concerns. Lollar points out that one area in which collaboration and interaction between public health and rehabilitation psychology may have substantial promise is that of the International Classification of Functioning, Disability and Health (ICF; World Health Organization, 2001). Rehabilitation psychology has been involved in the development of this tool for many years; the reader is advised to read the special section on the ICF in *Rehabilitation Psychology* published in 2005 (e.g., Bruyère & Peterson, 2005; Peterson, 2005) as well as an excellent compendium by Mpofu and Oakland (2010) for details of the ICF and its application.

EXAMPLES IN ACADEMIC INSTITUTIONS AND THE HEALTH CARE ARENA

Psychologists who train and/or supervise students, interns, and residents have an opportunity to encourage their trainees to effect change in other areas, multiplying the impact of the original trainer. Thus, integrating advocacy and consumer protection into the curriculum—as hoped for by Beatrice Wright (see earlier)—becomes all the more important. One relevant activity is advocating for board certification and other standards of quality in provision of professional services (Cox, 2010). Some faculties have begun either encouraging or requiring board certification of their professors. Key to being able to provide training is funding; Reid-Arndt, Stucky, Cheak-Zamora, DeLeon, and Frank (2010) overview federal graduate medical education funding and advocacy efforts involved in securing it. Psychologists in hospitals and other health care facilities have opportunities to advance the cause of consumer protection as well. Callahan

(2010) writes that rehabilitation psychologists are well situated to provide leadership in these arenas. He identifies competencies that rehabilitation psychologists have (clinical, analytical, relational, interventional, ethical, and financial) that position them as outstanding health care executives—thereby enabling increased influence in consumer protection and other areas.

The chapter on legal issues (Chapter 2) in this volume addresses some aspects of competency and capacity that are encountered in rehabilitation. It is incumbent on rehabilitation psychologists to protect the rights of those whose capacity may be diminished, weighing the need to provide care to individuals with limited ability to formulate educated decisions. A variety of roles in which a psychologist may find oneself and situations that give rise to assessment of capacity are described by Wood and Kubik (2005), including those of evaluator and educator of the courts.

One of the most elemental advocacy situations for a rehabilitation psychologist occurs when serving as a member of the rehabilitation team. Although it may seem unnecessary to be an advocate on a rehabilitation team, members of other disciplines may be unaware of psychological, familial, or other issues that can affect the patient's rehabilitation progress. Butt and Caplan (2010) note a number of problems occurring on treatment teams, including inadequate operational logistics, interpersonal conflicts, and lack of adequate psychological training among staff members. They describe the rehabilitation psychologist's role as advocate, educator, and team leader, as well as numerous other roles. Given the importance of the rehabilitation team in patient care, the advocacy role that rehabilitation psychologists take can have a significant impact on outcomes.

INVOLVEMENT IN THE POLITICAL PROCESS

Psychologists are often reluctant to become involved in politics, public policy, health insurance issues, and other such areas. However, these are areas that directly and significantly affect the field of psychology, as well as one's personal practice and the lives of our patients. It is essential to have a voice in the way that society creates and re-creates legislation, policy, and rules. The path is established by those who are heard; rarely do those who remain silent get what they desire. Involved psychologists can set the stage for the direction of the health care, the profession, patients' rights, and societal change.

There are many places one may learn about involvement in the political process. However, for some psychologists, participation may be limited due to time and/or financial resources. Means of becoming involved can include making political campaign contributions, volunteering to be involved in a campaign or other political process, or simply contributing to the political action committee (PAC) affiliated with one's state psychological association or special interest group. For others, becoming involved may include running for office oneself. Between the ends of the spectrum of minimal involvement and actually running for office, one may have an impact by contacting legislators about issues of concern, writing letters to the editor of local newspapers, and participating in community awareness activities as the opportunity arises. Another relatively simple, yet effective, way of becoming involved includes working through one's state psychological association and other interest groups.

INVOLVEMENT IN PROFESSIONAL ORGANIZATIONS

Remaining active and involved in various organizations is vital to staying abreast of the field and being able to facilitate improvements in larger scale patient care and professional issues. Rehabilitation psychologists are most often associated with the Division of Rehabilitation Psychology (Division 22) of the APA, and many are also members of Division 38 (Health Psychology) and Division 40 (Clinical Neuropsychology) and other divisions. There are myriad other organizations that focus more directly on specific disabilities (e.g., state and national brain injury, stroke, or spinal cord injury associations).

Often overlooked, yet critical to local change ("all politics are local"), are state psychological associations. Many psychologists seem unaware of the significance of their state psychological association in the legislative process as well as in other arenas. State psychological association leaders convene annually at a national meeting, the APA State Leadership Conference (SLC), where a significant part of the agenda includes education about effective advocacy (Sullivan, Newman, & Abrahamson, 2007). The conference focuses on four major areas of advocacy, identified as legislative, legal, marketplace, and public education. Many psychologists involved in the SLC over the years have been instrumental in advancing change in our field and society. The state psychological association played a significant role in getting the first state (Connecticut) to reform legislation to include mental health parity to do so (Abrahamson, Steele, & Abrahamson, 2003). E. Johnson (2007) summarized the role of the Business of Practice Network (BOPN), a group composed of psychologists from each state association, in advocating for psychologically healthy workplaces. Some state psychological associations have mentoring programs to facilitate educating psychologists about legislative issues and processes (Burney et al., 2009). Membership and active involvement in state psychological associations can be critical to advancing the agenda of psychology and those whom psychology serves.

Conclusion

Rehabilitation psychologists have an opportunity to influence the way that health care and other institutions affect the lives of individual patients, groups, and public policy. Serving as an advocate—in whatever forum is accessible and suits the individual psychologist—is an essential role; one may maintain that it is an obligation of the ethical professional.

Some psychologists argue that involvement in organizations comes at a cost—volunteer time and effort, actual dollars for dues and other expenses, and loss of income due to being away from one's office. Although true, it may well be that the cost of *not* being involved exceeds that of engaging in the process.

Short of involvement in organizations, political proceedings, and the like, the rehabilitation psychologist can assert positive influence on a frequent and ongoing basis by engaging in treatment that actively includes the elements of advocacy and consumer protection.

NINE

Intervention

As suggested by the name of the specialty, "interventions" of various sorts are fundamental and essential activities of rehabilitation psychologists in the service of helping to restore individuals with disabilities to satisfying and productive lives. Interventions have been described as "...activities that promote, restore, sustain, and/or enhance positive functioning and a sense of well-being in clients through preventive, developmental, and/or remedial services" (McHolland, Peterson, & Brown, 1987, pp. 163–164). Intervention competency was readily recognized as an important skill area by the National Council of Schools of Professional Psychology (NCSPP) when that organization began considering competency areas for curriculum in professional psychology (Bent & Cox, 1991). These authors found significance in the fact that the competency area was called *intervention* as opposed to *psychotherapy* in recognition of the increasing breadth of treatments provided by psychologists.

Although this description of intervention with recognition of its multiple and varied types was not specific to *rehabilitation* psychology, it may as well have been. The activities of rehabilitation psychologists in providing intervention build upon a strong clinical foundational skill set that is then applied to populations that generally do not present with *primary* psychological issues. Rather, most individuals treated in rehabilitation psychology have experienced physical injury, illness, or trauma (some with effects on cognitive function), and the psychological aspect of care is a *secondary consequence (albeit often one with pervasive effects)* of that physical fact. Certainly, individuals with primary psychological issues can and do sustain disabling injury, but a large percentage of persons in rehabilitation treatment likely have had no prior contact with psychologists or other mental health professionals. Rusin and Uomoto (2010, p. 259) noted: "Unlike most clinical psychologists, whose clients identify problems for which they actively seek help, the rehabilitation psychologist often treats patients who are psychologically naïve and sometimes unwilling to participate." This presents a unique set of challenges.

Part of the "intervention" role of the inpatient rehabilitation psychologist may be to *prepare* the patient and family for what is to come and why. This early education can foster a view of rehabilitation as a collaborative enterprise among patient, staff, and family, enhancing the likelihood of patient cooperation, and promote a sort of "informed participation" in treatment. Misgivings about engaging in psychological treatment and/or denial of the existence of any psychological or emotional concerns are common, perhaps most so among the psychologically inexperienced or uninformed. However, when the psychologist is introduced as a regular member of the team and psychological care that focuses on the *adjustment to physical change* is presented as a standard component of the program for every patient admitted to the unit (thereby "normalizing" psychological intervention), resistance to psychological services can be decreased.

Even when rehabilitation patients are willing participants in treatment, other factors often make intervention in this setting unique. Physical disability can, and often does, produce neurological impairment, speech and/or language deficits, and other cognitive and/or sensory losses that interfere with communication; these can hamper establishment of a therapeutic relationship and carryover of material from session to session (Rusin & Uomoto, 2010). Faced with patients exhibiting cognitive difficulties such as memory impairment or diminished awareness of deficit, the rehabilitation psychologist must be able to differentiate among an amnestic disorder, anosognosia, behavioral disturbance, and/or noncompliance with therapy, as the indicated interventions certainly differ as a function of the underlying cause(s) (Caplan, 2010; Ricker, 2010).

Factors that may interfere with psychological intervention in the acute stage of rehabilitation include the patient being medically/physically fragile, the demands of other therapies such as physical and occupational therapy, fatigue, medication side effects, sleep disturbance caused by unfamiliar surroundings, cognitive deficits, impaired awareness of deficit, and emotional issues that range from denial to apathy to extreme depression, anxiety, agitation, and avoidance.

Following an inpatient stay during which obstacles such as reluctance to engage in therapy, denial, and acute adjustment concerns have presumably diminished, the outpatient rehabilitation psychologist may find individuals and families to be more receptive to psychological services. By this time, the realities of the disability tend to be more readily appreciated, as the individual is confronted with social, environmental, and other obstacles to returning to a previous way of living. Intervention at this stage typically goes well beyond psychoeducational processes and support and may be more intense as the individual works to incorporate new physical, cognitive, emotional, and interpersonal realities into a revised self-concept that may entail significant modification of one's prior value hierarchy (Keany & Glueckauf, 1993; Wright, 1983).

As the practice of rehabilitation psychology requires diverse sets of knowledge and skills, it is not surprising that rehabilitation psychologists emerge from divergent education and training backgrounds (K. R. Thomas & Chan, 2000; but see Wegener, Hagglund, & Elliott, 1998, and Wegener, Elliott, & Hagglund, 2000, who argue the case for adhering to the Boulder model). Individuals from clinical psychology, counseling psychology, neuropsychology, and educational psychology, among other areas, find themselves drawn to the arena of rehabilitation. Furthermore, as impairments and disabilities treated by rehabilitation psychologists afflict people from all walks of life and virtually the entire age spectrum, diversity in practitioner training has some advantages for rehabilitation patients.

Given this diversity of background, training, and clinical populations, one would not expect a monolithic conceptualization of intervention. Indeed, the capacity to master and employ multiple means of intervention in a variety of contexts and situations is fundamental to competent practice in rehabilitation psychology (Cox, Hess, Hibbard, Layman, & Stewart, 2010). Interventions are expected to be suited to the needs of the individual, family, and/or system. In addition, assessment findings are to be integrated into the treatment planning and interventions being provided. The American Board of Rehabilitation Psychology (ABRP) Examiner Manual (ABRP, 2010, pp. 32–33) states:

> Successful Candidates provide interventions that involve a variety of treatment modalities (e.g., psychotherapeutic, behavioral and environmental interventions). Candidates select interventions appropriate to the needs of the client. Candidates integrate assessment findings (e.g., medical, psychosocial, psychometric results) into the treatment plan. In keeping with required Rehabilitation Psychology competencies, Candidates will demonstrate required therapeutic interventions as related to adjustment to disability, family/couples

therapeutic interventions related to adjustment to disability, behavioral management and sexual counseling with disabled populations.

Beatrice Wright, a pioneer in rehabilitation psychology, provided a framework of guiding principles for rehabilitation psychology (Wright, 1960, 1983), fundamental to which is the notion that the rehabilitation psychologist views an injury or illness as an *impairment,* as in the language of the International Classification of Functioning, Disability and Health (ICF; World Health Organization, 2001); functional consequences of that impairment are the *disability*; and barriers and disadvantages within society constitute the *handicap.* Viewing the individual as a part of this larger system, the rehabilitation psychologist provides and guides interventions intended to minimize handicaps, increase quality of life, and maximize individual functioning within the larger systemic framework. Thus, recommendations that arise from assessments or evaluations—and treatments that are provided—are not limited to person-centered ones; they frequently address the person–environment interaction or environment itself, including factors such as adaptive equipment, environmental accessibility, compensatory strategies, and recommendations for interpersonal/societal communication and interactions.

Given their inevitable interactions with the environment, individuals in rehabilitation cannot be treated in isolation. Minimization and/or prevention of handicap—the result of social barriers and other disadvantageous consequences of disability—are key aspects of rehabilitation psychology intervention. Thus, *prevention* is a cornerstone of *rehabilitation.* This became clear in the early days of rehabilitation psychology as psychologists attempted to articulate the parameters of the field (Wright, 1959). This aim can be construed to encompass secondary prevention of complications in persons with disabilities as well—for instance, assisting a stroke survivor to adhere to a treatment regimen that reduces the likelihood of a subsequent stroke or fostering compliance with a wheelchair push-up schedule aimed at avoiding development of pressure sores for a patient with paraplegia.

The interpersonal relationships of the patient as well as interactions with systems such as workplace, school, and community all are integral targets of intervention in rehabilitation psychology, as these are based on a biopsychosocial model that includes medical, psychological/emotional, cognitive, social, environmental, legal, and spiritual aspects of the individual's life (Rusin & Jongsma, 2001). Systems, broadly defined and ranging from the relationship of two individuals to the interaction of the individual with the community and society at large, are central considerations in planning and providing rehabilitation psychology interventions.

Furthermore, rehabilitation psychologists most frequently provide intervention and other services as part of a system of care. The team approach has enjoyed long-standing acceptance as the norm in rehabilitation, and psychologists have historically been considered "core" members of the treatment team (Butt & Caplan, 2010), although recent times have witnessed some fragmentation and modification of what constitutes a "team." "Psychological interventions" are provided directly by psychologists, but they are also offered by other health care professionals with psychologists serving a consultative role concerning such matters as motivation, treatment adherence, and the impact of cognitive deficits on therapeutic progress (see Chapter 7).

Rehabilitation psychology interventions are generally based on assessments that aid in identifying both preserved strengths and new-onset weaknesses; both types of information contribute to the development of treatment plans directed toward areas most in need of attention (Cox et al., 2010). Interested readers are referred to the assessment chapter (Chapter 6) in this book for more in-depth information about the roles and methods of assessment and their contributions to treatment planning. Assessment and evaluation-based interventions, including intermittent re-evaluations that document treatment progress and/or limiting factors, are an integral aspect of rehabilitation psychology.

Planning and provision of rehabilitation psychology interventions may be based on a theoretical or conceptual framework. However, treatment can also be driven simply by the phenomenology of the presenting problem. Rusin and Jongsma (2001) offered a guide to developing treatment plans for some two dozen psychological or neurobehavioral problems commonly encountered in rehabilitation settings (e.g., impulsivity, depression, memory impairment, neglect). For each item, they provide specific behavioral features; relevant *Diagnostic and Statistical Manual of Mental Disorders,* fourth edition (DSM-IV) diagnoses; suggested short-term and long-term goals; and an extensive list of possible therapeutic interventions. This practical, clinically oriented guide—which appeared before the explosion of interest in "evidence-based practice"—does not attempt to provide empirical support for efficacy of the suggested treatments, but rather offers recommendations grounded in clinical experience and a sizeable measure of common sense.

Rusin and Jongsma's (2001) book is an excellent source of foundations for treatment planning in rehabilitation for a variety of diagnoses and syndromes. Another useful reference (although not written from the perspective of rehabilitation psychology) is the second volume of *Handbook of Clinical Psychology Competencies* (J. C. Thomas & Hersen, 2010). Both books can serve as helpful guides to case conceptualization and treatment planning, using the diagnostic or symptom/syndrome-based model.

Intervention competency in rehabilitation psychology can be viewed through several lenses—as a function of medical diagnosis (e.g., stroke, brain injury, spinal cord injury), presenting problem (e.g., depression, anxiety, sleep disruption, poor motivation), setting (e.g., acute rehabilitation, rehabilitation hospital, outpatient clinic, private practice office, patient's home), modality of treatment (e.g., psychotherapy, pharmacotherapy, biofeedback, cognitive remediation, behavioral intervention, group or family therapy), and target of intervention (e.g., patient, family, staff, school, workplace, community). None of these are inherently correct or incorrect, nor does any single (or more than one) conceptualization capture all of the subtleties of the field. It is also clear that the models are not mutually exclusive.

Hibbard, Layman, and Stewart presented one conceptualization of rehabilitation psychology interventions that they refer to as the "**ABC**s of Rehabilitation Psychology Interventions" (Cox et al., 2010; Hibbard, Layman, & Stewart, 2010). The framework includes **A***djustment*, **B***ehavioral interventions*, and several "**C**s"—**C***ognitive remediation*, **C***ompensatory skills building*, and **C***onsultation and advocacy*. Although it does not correspond to the ABRP breakdown, we use this scheme to discuss some common interventions in rehabilitation psychology. Readers should note that, due to space constraints, the examples provided are meant to be illustrative, not exhaustive. Interested readers wishing more detailed treatments should consult two recent texts (Frank, Rosenthal & Caplan, 2010; Kennedy, 2012).

Adjustment

The majority of rehabilitation patients have experienced acute-onset changes that will be long-lived, if not permanent. The process of psychological adjustment to disability has been likened to the phases described in the dying patient (Kubler-Ross, 1969), and some early theorists (e.g., Siller, 1969) maintained that it was necessary for patients to progress through the proposed stages to achieve a satisfactory adjustment to their disability.

This perspective has been jettisoned in favor of a more flexible view that recognizes the importance and variability of, among other variables, both premorbid psychological factors and postmorbid emotional reactions. Although few would deny that the emotional states for which the stages are named (e.g., shock, depression, denial) do occur, it is well recognized that patients may have these reactions in any order, occasionally "backslide," skip a stage, and so forth. Caplan and Shechter (1987, p. 134) observed that "...the most helpful sort of stage theory may be the one that postulates the fewest stages—for example Prugh and Eckhardt's (1980) sequence of impact, recoil, and restitution—allowing the maximum explanatory power of individual differences (p. 134)."

Encouraging and promoting adjustment (or "accommodation") to disability is perhaps the key component of rehabilitation psychology practice. Therapy aimed at providing emotional support and education is a foundation and framework within which other interventions can be provided. It is within the context of adjustment that matters such as grief and loss, depression, anxiety, interpersonal relationships, and educational/vocational challenges are addressed. The importance of "supportive education" cannot be minimized, as the first step in learning to live with the "new normal" of acquired disability is understanding the medical facts and functional implications of one's condition. Absorbing this news is, of course, frequently distressing, so simultaneous provision of support, encouragement, and help in realistic "thinking through" of the future are tasks that frequently fall to the rehabilitation psychologist.

In formulating a treatment plan to foster adjustment, the skilled rehabilitation psychologist recognizes the relevance of many individual difference factors including the obvious ones of diagnosis, age, gender, cognitive ability, educational history, and work experiences but also more elusive and/or less well-studied factors such as the individual's spiritual orientation (Albright, Forcheimer, & Tate, 2010; Rippentrop, 2005) and cultural and ethnic identity (e.g., Arango-Lasprilla & Niemeier, 2007; Gallaher & Hough, 2001; Lomay & Hinkebein, 2006). Patients' emotional states are also likely to be affected by their prior experience (or lack thereof) with their particular condition, as this can shape their expectations about what the future holds. A person with a recent-onset stroke who has vivid memories of a grandparent with severe stroke-related deficits may feel demoralized and despairing, anticipating that same future. An individual with a new brain injury or spinal cord injury may have seen media reports (usually incompletely detailed) of cases of apparently miraculous recoveries from paralysis or coma and infer that he or she can achieve the same degree of improvement. If this does not occur, the emotional impact can be devastating.

A useful tactic that can help minimize patient frustration about progress that is always slower than one would wish is to help patients contrast their current abilities with those of several days or weeks ago (depending on the length of time since onset) instead of comparing current with pre-disability self. The latter comparison will almost always be depressing as it highlights "losses," whereas the shorter term contrast underscores gains made.

Recently, the concept of *patient resilience* has been explored in an effort to understand why some patients do not experience the high levels of distress seen in others (Quale & Schanke, 2010; White, Driver, & Warren, 2010). Despite the traditional view that loss or trauma is necessarily followed by grief or psychological distress, this is often not the case (Wortman & Silver, 1989), and to assume otherwise can lead to regrettable misunderstanding of the patient and his or her needs. Quale and Schanke (2010) suggest that absence of manifest psychological distress may not be a manifestation of denial but rather a resilient healthy coping response. They argue for the importance of providing this framework in psychoeducational programs for persons (and their families) following severe injury. This type of intervention fits the model of positive psychology (Ehde, 2010; Seligman, 1998; Seligman & Csikszentmihalyi, 2000), and interventions that focus on an individual's strengths as opposed to weaknesses (Cox & Sanders, 2002; White, Driver, & Warren, 2008) comports with the rehabilitation zeitgeist.

Given the central role of counseling among the services provided by rehabilitation psychologists, it is surprising that there is not more empirical evidence supporting its efficacy. There is a long tradition of studies of the incidence and "natural history" of emotional reactions to disability (e.g., Craig, Hancock, & Dickson, 1994; Kennedy & Rogers, 2000; Patterson et al., 1993), and other research has documented predictors and/or correlates of psychological outcomes of various sorts for both individuals with disabilities (e.g., deRoon-Cassini, St. Aubin, Valvano, Hastings, & Horn, 2009; Dryden et al., 2005; Elliott, Witty, Herrick, & Hoffman, 1991; Umlauf & Frank, 1983) and their caregivers (e.g., Alexander & Wilz, 2010; Davis et al., 2009; Gaugler, 2010; Perrin, Heesacker, Hinojosa, Uthe, & Rittman, 2009). However, the empirical support for the value of psychological intervention is not as substantial as one would hope.

Nonetheless, the "evidence-based landscape" is not barren. Some studies have shown that psychological intervention (with or without adjunctive pharmacological treatment) can reduce emotional distress and improve function in individuals with disabilities (e.g., Backhaus, Ibarra, Klyce, Trexler, & Malec, 2010; Hughes, Robinson-Whelan, Taylor, Swedlund, & Nosek, 2004; Kahan, Mitchell, Kemp, & Adkins, 2006). Kennedy, Duff, Evans, and Beedie (2003) reported diminished depression and anxiety in persons with spinal cord injury who participated in a coping effectiveness group training program. A recent evidence-based review concluded that cognitive-behavioral therapy was a promising treatment for emotional distress in persons with spinal cord injury (Mehta, et al., 2011). Wegener, Mackenzie, Ephraim, Ehde, and Williams (2009) found enhanced self-efficacy, improved mood, and fewer functional limitations among persons with amputations who participated in a group intervention program designed with this disability in mind. This comports with the findings of Pegg et al. (2005) that cognitively impaired persons with traumatic brain injury show greater improvements in function and more satisfaction as well as better effort in therapy when given personally relevant information about their condition compared to those who received more generic teaching.

Cognitive-behavioral therapy has met with some (Grober, Hibbard, Gordon, Stein, & Freeman, 1993) but not uniform (Lincoln & Flannaghan, 2003) success in treatment of depression after stroke. Pharmacological interventions also appear to have yielded mixed results (e.g., Hackett, Anderson, & House, 2005; Lauritzen et al., 1994), but a combination of prophylactic drug treatment and psychological intervention (L. S. Williams et al., 2007) offers hope of greater efficacy. As mentioned previously, psychological interventions with survivors of stroke or traumatic brain injury are hampered in many cases by the presence of aphasia, memory impairment, reduced awareness, or other higher cognitive disorders. Thus, this remains an area in need of further empirical exploration.

The previous discussion is clearly a limited one in both breadth and depth. The range of adjustment-related problems and situations for which the rehabilitation psychologist may be called upon to intervene is extensive, and even seasoned clinicians will require all of their varied skills and knowledge to work effectively in this setting. As a result, rehabilitation psychologists are rarely bored.

As caregivers play an important role in the lives of many rehabilitation patients after hospital discharge, some studies have examined methods of assisting caregivers to maintain their own health, both mental and physical. Schulz, et al. (2009) reported that caregivers of persons with spinal cord injury showed reductions in depression, feelings of burden, and health symptoms after participating in a "dual target" multicomponent program that offered education and supportive counseling to both caregiver and care recipient. Ipsen, Ravesloot, Arnold, and Seekins (2012) found reduced depression in caregivers of stroke survivors who participated in a web-based intervention, a methodology that is becoming more widely used, especially in rural areas where transportation to a hospital or doctor's office may be impractical.

Behavior

Interventions aimed at behavioral change may target issues such as social withdrawal, substance abuse (Bombardier & Turner, 2010), anger management (Hart et al., 2012), and poor motivation for and compliance with rehabilitation treatments. Although the following discussion focuses on behavior change in the patient, it should be recognized that, on occasion, the behavior that needs changing emanates from a team member or relative.

Behavior modification has a long history in rehabilitation psychology (Fordyce, 1982; Ince, 1976; Jacobs, 1993; Levenkron, 1987), using both operant and classical conditioning methods. Although other members of the treatment team may be familiar with the general concept of "behavior modification," it is typically the psychologist's responsibility to develop the specifics of a program for a particular individual (e.g., identifying target behaviors and triggers, specifying reinforcers and schedules, drawing up behavioral contracts). Fordyce (1982) noted four problem types that can be understood from a behavioral perspective: behavioral deficits, behavioral excesses, naturalistic punishment, and reinforcement of behavior. Space limitations preclude detailed illustrations of these forms and procedures for addressing them; we limit ourselves to one condition that, in some sense, served as a prototype for the use of behavioral methods in rehabilitation. Interested readers should consult the cited sources for examples of their application to such problems as anxiety, intemperate outbursts, inadequate personal hygiene, and poor compliance with prescribed treatments.

One of the earliest uses of behavior modification in rehabilitation was in the treatment of chronic pain. Recognizing how pain behavior could be shaped by the responses elicited from others, Fordyce (1976) outlined an operant approach to rehabilitation of chronic pain that involves the entire treating team. This multidisciplinary approach has become the accepted standard of care in numerous facilities. Among the "behavioral" features of this program was the understanding that analgesia administration in response to patient complaints of pain could create a strong learning effect in which pain relief is associated with medication. Over time, the patient learns to exhibit more "pain behaviors," justifying the request for more medication and potentially further increasing pain behavior and overt suffering. Making medication doses *time* contingent instead of *complaint* contingent both facilitates maintenance of a consistent (presumably effective) amount of medication and helps to eliminate the link between medication and pain relief.

Another behavioral aspect of this approach is the use of increasing quotas of exercise (rather than having the patient work until he or she began to hurt). Starting levels are set so as to be quite tolerable, followed by time-contingent, not pain-contingent, rest. Gradual increases in exercise are then implemented on a preplanned basis, circumventing the problem of patient pain level determining the level of activity. It should be added that, in addition to behavioral interventions, the psychologist can also offer counseling to promote self-efficacy and diminish catastrophizing reactions as well as relaxation training to improve pain tolerance.

The technique of motivational interviewing (Miller & Rolnick, 2002) has been increasingly employed with individuals with disabilities to encourage new, health-promoting behaviors as replacements for self-destructive ones. This may be especially effective in the rehabilitation setting, as recently injured patients can be particularly receptive if the disability-causing event resulted from their own risky behavior such as alcohol abuse (Bombardier & Rimmele, 1998).

Another domain where behavior change is often needed involves sexual function. Many disabling conditions have predictable consequences for sexual expression, and these typically require both teaching and counseling. Spinal cord injuries affect erectile ability and fertility in different ways depending on the level and completeness of the lesion. Stroke and traumatic brain injury are often accompanied by impulsive behavior or neuropsychological deficits that can hamper the ability to communicate one's own needs or perceive signals from the partner.

With ever-shortening stays in rehabilitation, the subject of sexuality may be overlooked, as more pressing issues are felt to take precedence. Nonetheless, the seasoned rehabilitation psychologist will strive to ensure that patients and significant others have, at a minimum, a grasp of the impact of the disabling condition on sexual capacity and an understanding that the disability does not necessarily mean an end to one's sex life—that is, the topic of sex should be considered a live issue, another "activity of daily living." In achieving these two goals, the psychologist negotiates the first two phases of Annon's (1974) PLISSIT model of sexual counseling—giving Permission to discuss the subject and providing Limited Information. Working through the remaining phases (Specific Suggestions, Intensive Therapy) may not be needed with all patients, but when it is indicated it will usually occur after acute rehabilitation when interest in and opportunities for sexual expression tend to increase.

Biofeedback treatments are a form of behavior modification that require sophisticated training and equipment, but they have been used to great effect to improve movement of paretic limbs, reduce the effects of orthostatic hypertension, enhance motor control in persons with cerebral palsy (Brucker, 1984), and reduce chronic pain (Buckelew, et al., 1998).

The innovative method of constraint-induced movement therapy (CIMT) for paretic extremities derives from behavioral principles. Initially the subject of some controversy, as it appeared to be a punitive technique, CIMT has shown efficacy in improving motor function in affected limbs (Uswatte, Taub, Mark, Perkins, & Gauthier, 2010; Wolf, et al., 2006). The underlying idea is that individuals with right hemiplegia, for example, come to rely excessively on the intact limb, and whatever residual function may exist on the affected side is never tapped. By physically constraining the intact limb, the individual is forced to use (and thereby improve mobility and strength in) the affected side. Some questions remain about the long-term effects of CIMT (Sitori, Corbetta, Moja, & Gatti, 2010) and whether efficacy requires prolonged restraint (90% of waking hours) and highly intensive therapy (6 hours per day).

Cognition (and other Cs)

COGNITIVE REHABILITATION

Individuals who have experienced cognitive changes may benefit from learning cognitive remedial strategies through methods such as attention training (Sohlberg & Mateer, 2001) or instruction and practice in use of mnemonics and other memory enhancement strategies. Calendars, schedules, and notebooks may be of value, but external aids such as personal digital assistants and smartphones are assuming ever greater prominence in rehabilitation (Wilson & Kapur, 2008). "High tech" tools can be programmed to provide reminders, store information, offer step-by-step directions, and assist with other tasks in unobtrusive ways that are common among the able-bodied population. For this reason, they are often more easily accepted by rehabilitation patients who may well have had predisability experience with them. Clearly, the field has advanced a considerable distance beyond early efforts that were based largely on repetitive practice, with some attention devoted to trying to "train for generalization" beyond the trained task (e.g., Weinberg et al., 1977). Interested readers should consult the reviews by Cicerone and colleagues (2000, 2005, 2011), the chapters by Hart (2010) and Kirsch and Scherer (2010), the volumes by Stuss, Winocur, and Robertson (2008) and Eslinger (2002), and the numerous writings by Barbara Wilson (e.g., Wilson, 2002), as well as the journal *Neuropsychological Rehabilitation* established and edited by Wilson.

Eskes and Barrett (2009) proposed five categories of cognitive rehabilitation: (a) retraining of the impaired function; (b) optimization of preserved functions; (c) compensation through substitution of intact skills; (d) another form of compensatory technique based on use of environmental supports or devices; and (e) what they term "vicariation approaches," those that aim to recruit related unimpaired areas of the brain to take over responsibility for functions previously carried out by damaged areas. Selection of any one or more of these approaches will likely derive primarily from the results of assessment in the individual case.

Implementation may be the province of the rehabilitation psychologist, but speech therapists, occupational therapists, and a new class of "cognitive rehabilitation specialists" increasingly see this type of treatment as falling within their area of expertise. Collaboration among the various team members and consequent consistent reinforcement of strategy use across locations within the rehabilitation setting is desirable and may serve to promote generalization. This is an underlying principle of holistic cognitive rehabilitation pioneered by Ben-Yishay and colleagues (Ben-Yishay, Silver, Piasetsky, & Rattok, 1987) and further developed by Prigatano (1999).

An exciting development in cognitive rehabilitation has been the use of virtual reality (VR) technology, which allows the psychologist or other clinician to create approximations of real-world settings in cyberspace where patients can safely practice and rehearse new behavioral strategies, receiving precise feedback to help them modify their behavior to achieve desired aims. Schultheis and Rizzo (2001) provide a readable overview of work in this area and Rose, Brooks, and Rizzo (2005) reviewed VR applications for individuals with brain injury..

Cognitive rehabilitation may emphasize treatment of problems with higher cortical functions, but these deficits are almost invariably accompanied by difficulties in emotional, behavioral, familial, social, and/or vocational realms. Here again, the rehabilitation psychologist will need to draw on multiple clinical skills to provide the most effective services.

CONSULTATION

Treatment using a team approach is fundamental in rehabilitation (Butt & Caplan, 2010), whether multidisciplinary, interdisciplinary, or transdisciplinary, having evolved, at least in part, due to the complex needs of veterans following World War II and the Vietnam Conflict. The current wars in the Middle East have produced a disturbing increase in veterans surviving with multiple trauma (e.g., amputation and brain injury; burns and posttraumatic stress disorder), leading to establishment of several polytrauma centers devoted to multidisciplinary treatment of the multiple needs of these individuals. In some rehabilitation facilities, psychologists are leaders of the treatment team, and in others they are members of the "core" team, but at a minimum, psychologists serve as consultants to many other specialties. Indeed, it is the atypical rehabilitation psychologist that functions in isolation.

The topics or targets of consultation can span an immense range, encompassing identifying causes of poor motivation for therapy, assisting the team and patient in development of "behavioral contracts," advising nurses or therapists how to handle disinhibited behavior, collaborating with speech or occupational therapists in assessing cognitive functions, advising school personnel about need for likely accommodations for students resuming their education after brain injury, or serving a similar purpose for older individuals desiring to re-enter the workforce.

It is difficult to find empirically based literature supporting the value of the consultative role of the rehabilitation psychologist. This would be virtually impossible to investigate with adequate scientific controls. However, one can make a strong case for "face validity" in light of the profound psychological impact of many disabling conditions and the mounting evidence that distressed individuals do poorly with respect to long-term outcomes. A rehabilitation psychologist who is not in a position to offer one-on-one patient care (e.g., because of an unfavorable staff/patient ratio or inability to bill for this type of service) can still play a central role by discussing, analyzing, and advising about management strategies for problem behaviors displayed by patients (and family members); helping to resolve staff–patient conflicts; or teaching treatment team members psychologically informed ways of viewing and interpreting patient behaviors (Caplan & Shechter, 1993).

One of the few rehabilitation psychiatrists, Gans (1987) described a challenging but potentially fruitful consultative technique for dealing with problematic patient behaviors. The team-attended psychological interview (TAPI) is a three-part process involving initial presentation of biopsychosocial data and discussion by team members of what it feels like to work with the patient in question. This is followed by an interview of the patient viewed (and participated in) by the team (who may ask questions of the patient). The final part consists of a team discussion about and analysis of the psychological meaning of what they have heard in an effort to better understand the patient's situation and to formulate changes in the treatment plan. While TAPIs are likely to be logistically prohibitive in the current environment, the rehabilitation psychologist can nonetheless achieve some of the aims of the TAPI by formulating and then conveying to team members a richer view of "problem patients" and the genesis of their troubling behaviors than is likely to be gained by staff members working with the patient in isolation toward narrowly defined goals.

COMPENSATORY SKILL BUILDING

Learning to compensate for acquired limitations is a fundamental aim of many aspects of the rehabilitation process. This may involve substituting one way of achieving a behavioral goal for another means. Alternatively, entirely new skills may be learned. The following is an illustration of the latter.

Social skills training methods have an important role to play in rehabilitation, as those with new-onset disabilities will often benefit from learning concrete ways to respond to common reactions to disability displayed by able-bodied others in the community (stereotyped and/or demeaning responses that they themselves may well have shared in the prerehabilitation life). M. Dunn (1987) described a videotape (M. Dunn, Van Horn, & Herman, 1976) that he created (and starred in) illustrating both ineffective and adaptive reactions to situations such as being offered unwanted and unnecessary help or responding to questions about why one uses a wheelchair.

Due to legislative and policy mandates, rehabilitation psychologists working in inpatient settings are likely to see patients who fall into one of several specific diagnostic categories (Ashkanazi, Hagglund, Lee, Swaine, & Frank, 2010). To meet policy requirements to be classified as an inpatient rehabilitation facility, 75% of the admissions must fall into one of these categories: advanced osteoarthritis, amputation, brain injury, burns, congenital deformity, femur fracture, hip or knee replacement, multiple trauma, neurological disorders, polyarthricular rheumatoid arthritis, spinal cord injury, stroke, and systemic vasculitides.

The rehabilitation psychologist providing services on an inpatient unit may be required to be familiar with interventions that are beneficial in the relatively acute stages of these conditions—clearly a wide range of diagnostic categories. This will require knowledge of the medical aspects as well as the psychological issues that arise in relation to them. The aforementioned list of diagnostic categories is clearly based on *medical* or *physical* categorization and notably does not address psychological aspects as a primary concern. Effective intervention, however, includes attention to the psychological issues and the physical/medical issues *within the context of the demands and the regulatory requirements of the inpatient setting.*

Inpatient rehabilitation stays have shortened over the years, and the intervention role of the inpatient rehabilitation psychologist tends to be that of focusing on acute adjustment, recognition of issues that arise, and treatment planning for future care. Treatment of anxiety and depression is high on the list of the problems to which rehabilitation psychologists attend in an inpatient setting. These factors may be so extreme as to limit patients' level of participation and active engagement in other therapies (e.g., physical therapy). Given the requirement for active participation in rehabilitation efforts, a patient is no longer permitted to stay on a rehabilitation unit for long when not engaged in treatment. Thus, the ability of the psychologist to intervene in such cases, acting as part of the therapeutic team with other health care professionals, may facilitate active treatment on a unit from which the patient may otherwise be discharged.

Conclusion

It is doubtful that any psychological specialty surpasses rehabilitation psychology in the range of medical conditions, psychosocial and familial problems, environmental factors, and systemic issues confronted on a daily basis. The range of knowledge and skills required to work effectively with the many and varied "players" is equally broad. This chapter can only provide a bit of the flavor of the work of rehabilitation psychologists as they endeavor to assist persons with disabilities in establishing (or re-establishing) satisfying and meaningful lives.

TEN

Science Base and Knowledge

As with virtually all health care specialties, there is increasing pressure on rehabilitation psychology practitioners to proffer empirical evidence for the efficacy and cost efficiency of their work. Fortunately, this particular psychological specialty is better equipped than many others to meet that challenge, in large part because of two related historical emphases in rehabilitation: (a) the need to demonstrate "change" in treated patients, that is, that therapy (occupational therapy, physical therapy, speech therapy, or psychological therapy) produces improvement in patients' abilities to manage real-world tasks, and (b) measurement of functional outcome. Rehabilitation facilities whose patients did not benefit from therapy and achieve worthwhile outcomes would not have survived, as insurance carriers would not long have paid for their services.

Rehabilitation psychologists absorbed these aspects of the "rehabilitation zeitgeist" and applied their knowledge and techniques accordingly. For example, psychologists have been at the forefront of the development of many outcome measures (Heinemann & Mallinson, 2010), ensuring the inclusion of emotional, cognitive, and social components, in addition to helping to refine their psychometric properties and practicality of the measures (see Tate, 2010, for a comprehensive collection of outcome measures applicable to brain injury). Also, neuropsychologists working in rehabilitation settings frequently found that staff, patients, and family members had little or no interest in their diagnostic acumen, a skill that became increasingly obsolete with the advent and refinement of neuroimaging techniques. Instead, rehabilitation neuropsychologists learned the importance of inferring from test performances which types of therapeutic interventions offered the greatest chances of success, in this way becoming close collaborators with speech therapists, occupational therapists, and physical therapists (e.g., Wertheimer et al., 2008).

Rehabilitation psychologists also came to recognize the importance of using test data to make informed predictions and recommendations about daily life activities after hospital discharge, advising patients and families about desirable safety measures, vocational or educational options (e.g., Miller & Donders, 2003), financial management (Hoskin, Jackson, & Crowe, 2005), and driving, among other topics. (NB: It should be noted that a substantial body of literature on prediction of driving after neurological injury using neuropsychological tests produced a raft of partially overlapping findings and recommendations. Newer tests—such as the "driving scenes" subtest of the Neuropsychological Assessment Battery [Brown et al., 2005] or technology such as virtual reality [Schultheis & Mourant 2001] may prove more reliable and "ecologically valid.") Initially, of course, these inferences and advice were only educated guesses, as no data existed showing the predictive validity of neuropsychological tests for activities of daily living. In recent years, however, clinician-researchers have placed greater emphasis on studying the association of neuropsychological assessment results with aspects of functional outcome.

The authors of an early article (Heaton & Pendleton, 1981) posited that performance on complex neuropsychological tests ought to predict overall functional outcome, and scores on more focused tasks should predict patients' capacity to perform discrete daily life functions. Fifteen years later, although one study (Bowman, 1996) had found "a modest but meaningful level of predictive utility…for occupational and activity functioning using neuropsychological, demographic, and emotional variables" (p. 391), contributors to the volume by Sbordone and Long (1996) still had to acknowledge that "…the ecological validity of most specific measures has yet to be established" (Cubic & Gouvier, 1996, p. 220) and that the move toward "…more ecologically valid tests of personality and behavior has barely begun" (Judd & Fordyce, 1996, p. 348).

Laments about the limited study of ecological validity of neuropsychological tests are now somewhat less justified (Chaytor & Schmitter-Edgecombe, 2003). For example, Novak, Sherer, and Penna (2010) reviewed studies demonstrating the value of test data in predicting return to work and driving, decision-making capacity, and need for supervision. A recent volume (Marcotte & Adams, 2010) on the neuropsychology of daily life functioning ranges widely across diagnostic categories (e.g., traumatic brain injury, multiple sclerosis, human immunodeficiency virus [HIV]-associated cognitive decline, sports injuries) and functions (e.g., driving, adherence to medication regimens, vocational capacity). Notably, virtually none of the contributors to this volume are strongly identified with rehabilitation psychology, but their work speaks directly to the concerns and needs of rehabilitation clinicians.

Rehabilitation psychologists have functioned as exemplary scientist-practitioners, endeavoring to base clinical activities on empirical data in accordance with Standard 2—Competence—of the American Psychological Association (APA) Ethical Code. Interested readers are urged to review the special issue of *Rehabilitation Psychology* edited by Chwalisz and Chan (2008) on research design, methodology, and statistical analysis as applied in rehabilitation settings. The articles in that issue (as well as others, e.g., Enders, 2011) describe some of the best scientific principles and practices of the field, providing information that practitioners should absorb and use in critiquing new research in their quest for the most useful and well-validated clinical techniques.

Just as the clinical value of good empirical data is indisputable, so too is the importance of sound conceptual models and theories. Indeed, most readers have probably heard the quote (often attributed to Kurt Lewin, a spiritual grandfather of rehabilitation psychology, as much of the early theoretical work in the field grew out of Lewin's writings): "There is nothing so practical as a good theory." In recognition of the need for balance between data and concepts, the central journal for the field—*Rehabilitation Psychology*—publishes articles describing both theoretical models (e.g., Chronister & Chan, 2006; Leibowitz & Stanton, 2007) and constructs such as resilience (Catalano, D., Chan, F., Wlson, L., Chiu, C-Y., & Muller, V., 2011; White, Driver, & Warren, 2008) and hope (Kortte, Sevenson, Hosey, Castillo, & Wegener, Snyder, Lehman, Kluck, & Monsson, 2006), as well as systematic literature reviews (e.g., Gaugler, 2010). These works will likely spur additional empirical studies of these and other concepts, further enlarging the database supporting the contributions of rehabilitation psychology to clinical practice. In addition, the journal has provided tutorials on some of the more sophisticated analytic techniques (e.g., Jackson, 2010).

In brief, we endorse the view of Sexton, Hanes, and Kinser (2010) in their discussion of the process of translating science into practice that the two are inextricably linked and that we need to emphasize the hyphen in the phrase "scientist-practitioner." These authors note that science and practice are "…two sides of a different coin: each bringing a unique perspective to understanding the same process of client change" (p. 154).

Some Barriers to Rehabilitation Research

It must be acknowledged that research in rehabilitation settings presents some unique and difficult challenges. First, the desired level of experimental control is typically not possible. Patients are invariably involved in multiple daily therapies, and the content of these is individualized on the basis of patient needs; this makes it difficult to tease apart the relative impacts of specific interventions. Whyte and Hart (2003) have addressed this problem, suggesting that a "levels of analysis" approach can enhance the researcher's ability to identify unique effects of particular treatments. Hart (2009), too, has thoughtfully addressed the multiple problems of defining "treatment," noting that researchers must consider both the content of treatment and the processes by which it is delivered and through which it causes change. "The great diversity of rehabilitation settings, populations, and targeted outcomes of treatment, from nerve and muscle function to participation in social roles, further contributes to the lack of uniform definition of interventions" (p. 625).

Second, it is difficult, if not impossible, to "mask" the identity of members of an experimental group, as they will likely be receiving an intervention not offered to those in the control group.

Third, researchers must decide how any control group(s) should be managed. Hart, Fann, and Novack (2008) provide a detailed analysis of the factors to consider when deciding whether the control group should receive, for example, no treatment, delayed treatment, or routine care.

A fourth challenge to rehabilitation research concerns the considerable individual variability within injury/illness categories. No two brain injuries, strokes, spinal cord injuries, cases of multiple sclerosis, and so forth are alike. "Lesion groups" can be created based on primary locus of injury, but these will lack purity of the sort one can obtain in studies of induced lesions in laboratory animals. The presence of comorbid conditions also complicates creation of uniform groups, whether these conditions are purely physical in nature (e.g., spinal cord injury coexisting with other fractures) or a mix of physical and psychological (posttraumatic stress disorder and brain injury). As pointed out by Barnett et al. (2012), some rehabilitation patients have low-incidence conditions, hampering efforts to secure a sufficient number of individuals to carry out a randomized controlled trial (RCT).

Fifth, many conditions treated in rehabilitation settings are characterized by some degree of recovery. Therefore, unless treatment is begun after it has been established that natural recovery has clearly plateaued, it can be difficult to disentangle the effects of intervention from those attributable simply to the passage of time and the natural history of the condition.

A sixth obstacle involves the ethics of withholding of potentially useful treatment from a control group. One can, of course, argue that until a treatment has been conclusively demonstrated to be effective, there is no ethical issue in providing treatment to only the "experimental" group. However, in testing the efficacy of a treatment, one presumably has some a priori reason (or perhaps even pilot data) suggesting that it merits formal investigation, in which case that "agnostic" position becomes difficult to maintain.

A seventh impediment to research in rehabilitation is the potential conflict between the goals of the researcher and those of the patients/participants. The latter naturally wish to devote their time to therapeutic activities that will enhance their function, whereas the former seek to capture therapy time in the service of advancing science. There is also the desirability of limiting the influence on the research outcome under investigation of what, in the researcher's eyes, are extraneous variables; this could mean withholding of other therapies, an approach fraught with ethical problems.

A Partial Solution

In light of these and other obstacles, it is not surprising that what is typically considered the "gold standard" of research design—the RCT—is a relatively *rara avis* in rehabilitation. It should be noted, however, that Perdices, Schultz, Tate, McDonald, and Togher (2006) have cited evidence that the methodological quality of RCTs has been overrated, and B. Williams (2010) observed that results of RCTs may often be inapplicable to individual patients. Code (2000) opined that RCTs of aphasia therapy are poorly suited to address questions of everyday clinical management. Furthermore, the charge often levied at single-subject designs (SSDs)—that they offer limited generalizability—also applies to RCTs in the view of B. Williams (2010). He observed that only certain subsets of participants in an RCT will benefit from treatment, and the results will not typically specify which participants (with which particular characteristics) improve, thereby offering little value to the practitioner faced with a series of "$N = 1$" cases. Also, RCTs may report statistically significant—albeit clinically modest—results by virtue of having a large sample. As B. Williams noted: "...such a result may have limited predictive utility at the level of the individual patient" (p. 109).

The following brief on behalf of single-subject research designs should not be misconstrued as a simultaneous denigration of RCTs, as the latter clearly have an important role to play in scientific research. But for the previously detailed obstacles, no doubt RCTs would be more common in the rehabilitation psychology literature.

In light of these factors, certain advantages of the intensive case study approach become apparent. Indeed, Perdices and Tate (2009) argued that SSDs have been seriously undervalued by many investigators and opined that they "…fit hand-in-glove with day-to-day clinical practice…" (p. 905). Readers are urged to consult the chapter by Freeman and Lim (2010) for a sophisticated discussion of the skills and knowledge required to carry out competent single-subject research. They argue that such methods "…can also be used to assist practitioners in determining the impact of their efforts" (p. 421). What could be more "rehabilitation relevant"?

Historically considered a "poor relation" with respect to methodology, the intensive investigation of individual cases ("single case experimental designs" is the phrase used by Tate et al., 2008) has played an increasingly important role in rehabilitation. Indeed, Perdices et al. (2006) surveyed the methodology of entries in the Psychological Database of Brain Impairment Treatment Efficacy and found single case designs to be the most prevalent form.

A considerable degree of methodological rigor has developed for "$N = 1$" studies. Tate et al. (2008) devised an 11-item evaluative scale for assessing the quality of single case designs that includes factors such as identification of clearly defined, measurable target behaviors; adequate establishment of baseline behavior; and interrater reliability of observations of target behaviors. Perdices et al. (2006) asserted: "Sophisticated SSDs incorporating, among other things, multiple baselines across subjects and behaviours, as well as randomization of the order of active treatment phases can, potentially, provide a level of evidence with the hierarchy of EBCP (evidence-based clinical practice) comparable to that of RCT's" (p. 130). Callahan and Barisa (2005) reviewed the analytic technique of statistical process control for single cases. Meta-analytic analyses of SSDs are also possible (Robey, Schulz, Crawford, & Sinner, 1999).

As the fundamental question in rehabilitation is whether the particular patient is benefitting from treatment, it is important to be able to establish the impact of interventions apart from improvement due to natural recovery. Perdices (2005) offers a concise discussion and illustration of three methods of demonstrating clinically significant change in individual cases originally proposed by Jacobson, Follette, and Revenstorff, (1984) and also touches on the calculation of the "reliable change index" applicable to individual patients.

In SSDs, patients can serve as their own controls; one need not be concerned, for example, with trying to "match site and extent of lesion across groups." One can modify the treatment protocol as one proceeds and develop new tests to address phenomena of interest. Practitioners in the field of cognitive neuropsychology (whose best work often appears in the journal of that name) have offered numerous elegant, detailed, and provocative accounts of "$N = 1$" assessment and intervention.

Illustrations of Rehabilitation Psychology's Evidence Base

A comprehensive treatment of the evidence base of rehabilitation psychology practice exceeds the scope of this chapter. Furthermore, readers will find many relevant empirical studies described in the chapters dealing with the major domains of practice. Therefore, we provide in the following sections some illustrative examples of empirical justification for various activities of contemporary rehabilitation psychologists using as an organizing scheme certain functions designated as "essential" by the American Board of Rehabilitation Psychology.

Adjustment to Disability: Patient and Family

Historically, this has been the primary area in which rehabilitation psychologists provided clinical services. One would hope to find substantial empirical evidence that effective psychological treatment fosters better outcome, but the supporting data are not as numerous and compelling as would be desired. One might also anticipate finding a solid evidentiary base demonstrating that those rehabilitation patients who exhibit resilience in response to disability have better outcomes than those whose progress is compromised by depression, anxiety, or other negative emotional states. The discussion by White, Driver, and Warren (2008) makes clear that this is an area of great potential applicability to rehabilitation populations, but one that requires much further study. However, there is some evidence that survivors of spinal cord injury who exhibit positive affect experience higher levels of subjective well-being than those who do not (Kortte, Gilbert, Gorman, & Wegener, 2010). A similar facilitating effect of an "active approach" on quality of life and functional ability was seen in individuals who sustained complex musculoskeletal injuries in automobile accidents (Hall, Marshall, Mercado, &Tkachuk, 2011). Furthermore, in a study of stroke survivors, Seale, Berges, Ottenbacher, and Ostir (2010) found that increases in positive emotions were associated with improved functional status.

A recent (February 2010) special section in *Rehabilitation Psychology* contained several articles describing the functional effects of patient resilience and positive mood in rehabilitation populations (deRoon-Cassini, Mancini, Rusch, & Bonanno, 2010; Kortte, Gilbert, Gorman, & Wegener, 2010; Quale & Schanke, 2010; Seale, Berges, Ottenbacher, & Ostir, 2010; White, Driver, & Warren, 2010). These works also provide further evidence against the inevitability of stage theories that mandate a period of depression as the gateway to "adjustment."

"Adjustment" varies over time in many rehabilitation populations (e.g., Seale, Berges, Ottenbacher, & Ostir, 2010) and among family members, especially those who are called upon to provide care. The relatively sheltered environment of the rehabilitation unit may shield some patients from full confrontation with their new limitations, whereas exposure to the real world after discharge can induce grieving, frustration, and depression. Also, caregivers can't truly fathom the extent of their new responsibilities until after their loved one returns home. Thus, it is not surprising to learn that caregivers of stroke survivors have been reported to experience sizable shrinkage in the areas of personal relationships, work, and avocational activity (Rochette, Desrosiers, Bravo, Tribble, & Bourget, 2007).

Another factor contributing to the dynamic of adjustment is a diminishing degree of anosognosia in certain groups. Although it might be expected that more accurate self-awareness would lead to increased distress as one's losses become more apparent, this is not invariably true. Malec and Moessner (2000) reported that individuals who participated in an outpatient brain injury treatment program showed both improved awareness and reduced emotional distress, and both factors were associated with positive behavioral outcomes.

Some investigations have shown that depression impedes progress in rehabilitation and limits functional and social outcome (e.g., van Wijk, Algra, van de Port, Bevaart, & Lindeman, 2006). Among stroke survivors, depression even appears to place one at greater risk of death (Jorge, Robinson, Arndt, & Starkstein, 2003; L. Williams, Ghose, & Swindle, 2004), and treatment with a combination of antidepressants and patient and family education and counseling (L. S. Williams et al. 2007) or medication coupled with problem-solving therapy (R. Robinson et al., 2008) enhances outcome. The possibility of preexisting depression should be considered, as this may have negative implications for post–hospital discharge destination (Nuyen, et al., 2007). Although S. Thomas and Lincoln (2008) found that expressive language impairment and level of disability predicted poststroke depression in the first 6 months, Hackett and Anderson (2005) concluded from their systematic review that research results are not yet sufficiently consistent to permit accurate prediction of poststroke depression so that interventions could be most efficiently targeted.

Dreer, Elliott, Shewchuck, Berry, and Rivera (2007) observed that caregivers of persons with spinal cord injury experienced depression at a rate comparable to that of persons with spinal cord injury themselves. Depression, subjective sense of burden, and duration of caregiving were identified as predictors of accidents among caregivers of persons surviving a stroke (Hartke, King, Heinemann, & Semik, 2006). Clearly, injured caregivers cannot continue to provide effective care. In a study of burden among caregivers of people with traumatic brain injury 1 year after injury, Davis et al. (2009) identified the importance of the caregiver's own medical/psychiatric history, coping styles, and perceived social support as determinants of perceived burden, leading them to call for stress management intervention to be offered prophylactically to caregivers as a means of fostering better long-term outcome for the injured person.

Grant, Elliott, Giger, and Bartolucci (2001) reported that social support was associated with life satisfaction among caregivers of stroke survivors. Furthermore, social problem-solving ability was linked with both caregiver depression and health, findings with certain treatment implications, as targeted therapy has been shown to improve features of problem-solving abilities (Nezu, Nezu, & Perri, 1989). The evidence that caregivers of older persons with stroke (Berg, Palomaki, Lonnqvist, Lehtihalmes, & Kaste, 2005) and those with impaired expressive language (Blonder, Langer, Pettigrew, & Garrity, 2007) are at increased risk for depression offers a basis for justifying preventive measures such as psychological counseling. The crisis intervention approach of Palmer, Glass, Palmer, Loo, and Wegener (2004) constitutes one potentially fruitful tactic.

In view of the importance of the caregiver role, it is regrettable that Visser-Meily, Post, Riphagen, and Lindeman (2004) concluded from their review of some 45 measures of caregiver burden that, although most exhibited good internal consistency and validity, little was known about their responsiveness to change, and the authors concluded that no single measure could be recommended above the others. Clearly, further work is needed in this area, preferably multicenter studies that might arrive at a consensus measure.

In thinking about "adjustment to disability," one should not lose sight of the (possibly surprising) fact that acquired disability may have positive effects. McMillen and Cook (2003) found that individuals with spinal cord injury interviewed 18 to 36 months after onset reported increased compassion and closer family relations in addition to diminished alcohol consumption. For further general discussion of the topic of posttraumatic growth, readers should consult Tedeschi and Calhoun (2004), and those interested in its relevance to brain injury should see the article by McGrath and Linley (2006).

Assessment

Readers will find much of the empirical support for major aspects of assessment in rehabilitation psychology in the assessment chapter (Chapter 6) of this text. Here we touch on a few assessment-related topics.

The decreasing average length of stay for inpatient rehabilitation has been accompanied by an even greater emphasis on efficiency, especially at the point of initial assessment, as there is pressure to move on to the *raison d'etre* of rehabilitation—intervention. This is why reliable and valid screening tests such as the Repeatable Battery for the Assessment of Neuropsychological Status (Randolph, 1998), a cognitive assessment instrument that offers the advantage of multiple forms, permitting serial testing that can document progress in rehabilitation, are desirable. However, as discovered by Wilde (2006), the factor structure of assessment measures obtained with neurologically intact participants may differ from that found when they are used with common rehabilitation populations such as persons with stroke or traumatic brain injury; thus, interpretive caution is necessary.

As noted previously, once their diagnostic services became largely superfluous with the refinement of modern imaging procedures, rehabilitation neuropsychologists gravitated in the direction of establishing ecological validity of existing tests and developing new measures with predictive value for daily life tasks. Hoskin, Jackson, and Crowe (2005) developed a 13-item Money Management Survey (MMS) to be completed by case managers of individuals with traumatic brain injury; the instrument inquired about matters such as failure to preserve money for essentials, impulsive spending, and failure to pay bills on time. The authors found that neuropsychological test performance showed modest predictive value for overall score on the MMS, but prediction of specific financial behaviors was more accurate.

One relatively unique aspect of assessment in rehabilitation psychology is the frequent need to rely on collateral reports, as for certain groups (e.g., those with stroke or traumatic brain injury) there may be doubt about their ability to provide reliable responses (Toedter et al., 1995); excluding these individuals would skew a research sample in the direction of more intact or well-functioning participants and therefore be unrepresentative. Reports from significant others may also be of value as a comparative standard in assessing accuracy of the patient's self-perception. Clinicians must be aware of factors that could influence honesty of report; for instance, if drug or alcohol use is at issue, self-reports may tend toward the temperate, and patient–proxy agreement may be low (Sander, Witol, & Kreutzer, 1997), while greater consensus may be found for matters like participation in community activities (Hart et al., 2010). However, even as benign an inquiry as one related to ambulation may produce disparities in patient and collateral ratings (Powell, Johnston, & Johnston, 2007).

If patients are to benefit from rehabilitation, one expects that they should see the need for it and be active participants. Individuals with either neurologically based anosognosia or psychologically based "denial" or "minimization" may fail to acknowledge their new limitations and therefore not see the need for therapy. As mentioned earlier, comparison of patient and proxy reports offers one means of gauging level of awareness, and formal instruments have been devised for this purpose. For example, the Awareness Questionnaire (Sherer Bergloff, Boake, High, & Levin, 1998) consists of three forms, one each to be completed by the patient, relative, and clinician, respectively; items involve comparing current abilities to those prior to injury or illness and giving ratings on a 5-point scale ("much worse" to "much better").

Many individuals who are well aware of their disability may exhibit "avoidant coping" (Lazarus & Folkman, 1984) in the form of minimal participation in therapy, behavior that augurs poorly for rehabilitation progress (Lenze et al., 2004). (It should be noted, however, that compliance may be "situation specific," and compliance in different situations may be associated with different measures of outcome;(Schoenberger, Humle, Zeeman, & Teasdale, 2006.) Early identification of those in need of more than the usual amounts of support and encouragement could foster improved outcomes. Kortte, Veiel, Batten, and Wegener (2009) detected good psychometric properties and solid correlations of an index of avoidance (the Acceptance and Action Questionnaire; Hayes et al., 2004) with measures of mood, hope, and spiritual well-being in addition to good predictive validity for satisfaction with rehabilitation as well as satisfaction with life and functional status at 3-month follow-up.

Intervention

Some aspects of the impact of rehabilitation psychology treatment are briefly considered for psychological and cognitive factors, respectively. Further discussion of scientific support for rehabilitation psychology interventions is found in the intervention chapter (Chapter 9) of this text. Although not offering an empirical evidence base, a good practical resource is the "treatment planner" by Rusin and Jongsma (2001) that addresses numerous clinical problems commonly encountered in rehabilitation settings (e.g., depression, sexual acting out, denial, emotional lability) and offers detailed management suggestions.

Pegg et al. (2005) showed that patients with traumatic brain injury who were given personalized information about their condition (e.g., through individualized discussion about their injuries, test results, progress in therapy, discharge plans, etc.) showed better effort in therapy, made more progress, and were more satisfied with the rehabilitation experience than were patients who received only generic discussion sessions. Backhaus, Ibarra, Klyce, Trexler, and Malec (2010) reported greater perceived self-efficacy (PSE) in persons with brain injury and their caregivers who participated in a cognitive-behavioral therapy (CBT) group compared to controls. These authors propose that PSE be viewed as a target for intervention, improvement in which could enhance factors traditionally viewed as indices of "adaptation" after brain injury such as psychological well-being and quality of life. After reviewing studies of CBT offered to persons with spinal cord injury, Mehta, et al. (2011) concluded that the treatment is a promising one for persons with SCI experiencing depression, anxiety and difficulty coping. They note that CBT is a multifactorial approach and that further research is needed to identify the element(s) with the greatest therapeutic impact.

Rath, Simon, Langenbahn, Sherr, and Diller (2003) reported improved problem-solving abilities among outpatient brain injury survivors who underwent an innovative training program that taught strategies targeting emotional self-regulation and logical thinking deficits. In a more recent contribution, Rath, Hradil, Litke, and Diller (2011) offer a concise overview of their conceptualization of impairments in problem-solving behavior in survivors of acquired brain injury (ABI), summarize some relevant research, and provide concrete examples of certain maladaptive assumptions, beliefs, and expectations exhibited by persons with ABI along with suggestions for interventions in such cases,

Hackett, Anderson, and House (2005) used the Cochrane method to analyze studies of antidepressant treatment in stroke survivors, concluding that routine use was not supported. An updated review (Hackett, Anderson, House, & Xia, 2009) reached a modified conclusion that antidepressants should be used with caution after stroke in light of the relatively small therapeutic effects and troubling incidence of adverse events. From the small number of relevant studies available for review, they concluded that psychotherapy alone was not an effective treatment for poststroke depression once it is present. However, a related review of studies of prevention (Hackett, Anderson, House, & Halteh, 2009) suggested that psychotherapy had a modest positive impact on mood and in the prevention of depression. The authors opined that further investigation is warranted of the effect of education, advice, and problem-solving therapies in the management of stroke survivors. There is also a need for studies examining the impact of novel psychological interventions such as the "crisis intervention" approach described by Palmer, Glass, Palmer, Loo, and Wegener (2004).

Although most rehabilitation treatments are delivered by trained professionals, a broader approach that includes the family in a therapeutic role may be efficacious as well. Braga, DePaz, and Ylvisaker (2005) studied children with traumatic brain injury who were treated for 1 year either by clinicians or by family members who had been trained to deliver therapy embedded in routine daily life activities. Although both groups improved on measures of physical and cognitive functioning, only the family-treated participants achieved significant—and clinically meaningful—degrees of improvement. Clearly, the potential burden on the family and the difficulties that may accompany having to manage dual roles (both therapist and parent) must be considered in devising any such intervention.

In certain instances, the most practical and/or useful target of intervention is not the patient or family members but the treating staff. Temple, Zgaljardic, Yancy, and Jaffray (2007) described the positive impact of a crisis intervention program for staff members of a residential brain injury rehabilitation unit. Following training, participants reported increased comfort in dealing with difficult patient behaviors.

With respect to interventions for cognitive deficits, there has been a true paradigm shift and explosion of research in this area in the past 20 years. Many publications provide detailed analyses of single cases (e.g., Svoboda & Richards, 2009, on treatment of a patient with severe anterograde amnesia) or small groups (e.g., Lengenfelder, Chiaravalloti, & DeLuca, 2007, who taught self-generation strategies to people with memory deficits following traumatic brain injury; Frassinetti, Angeli, Meneghello, Avanzi, & Ladavas, 2002, who demonstrated enduring reduction of unilateral neglect with the use of prismatic lenses). Three literature reviews by Cicerone and colleagues (2000, 2005, 2011) and articles by Barrett et al. (2006) and by Bowen and Lincoln (2007) on treatment of neglect and by Cicerone, Levin, Malec, Stuss, and Whyte (2006) on interventions for executive dysfunction, as well as the broader overviews in the chapter by Hart (2010) and the volumes by Wilson (2002), Wilson, Herbert, and Shiel (2003), and Johnstone and Stonington (2009), offer good summaries for the interested reader.

Adaptive/Assistive Technology

This area has seen explosive growth in recent years with the rapid development of microtechnology, creating smaller, more user-friendly (and wallet-friendly) devices to help individuals compensate for a variety of disabilities. For example, an early report by Wilson and colleagues (Wilson, Emslie, Quirk, & Evans, 1999) described use of a paging system to provide reminders to perform certain activities to an individual with traumatic brain injury–related memory impairment. This intervention enabled the user to live virtually independently, despite his limitations. Kirsch et al. (2004) developed a means of delivering at fixed intervals via a personal digital assistant the reminder "be brief" to a young man with socially disabling hyperverbosity. The intervention was effective as long as the cues remained in place. Kirsch and Scherer (2010) discuss relevant issues of problem identification, choice of intervention technique, and parameters for most effectively pairing person and technology.

Continuing miniaturization of components coupled with increasing capacity of computer chips will no doubt support further growth of "high tech" interventions employing personal computers, smartphones, virtual reality (VR), and other tools to help cognitively impaired individuals ameliorate the impact of their difficulties on daily life activities. Schultheis and Rizzo (2001) provide a useful review of VR-based neuropsychological rehabilitation for several forms of higher cortical dysfunctions and for rehearsing daily life tasks such as cooking and driving. The paper by Rizzo, Schultheis, Kerns, and Mateer (2004) offers a detailed look at the advantages of VR. A most practical application of VR is found in the report by Katz, Ring, Naveh, Kizony, Feintuch, and Weiss (2005), who described the use of VR to teach safe street crossing to stroke survivors with unilateral neglect.

Social Psychology of Disability

There is a large and varied literature dating back to the early days of the field dealing with negative perceptions and social stereotypes concerning persons with disabilities. D. Dunn (2010) provides an eloquent treatment of the impact of social factors on the disability experience, citing both theory and research in support of Myerson's (1948) view that "...the problems of the handicapped are not physical but social and psychological" (p. 2). The literature emphasizes the attitudes and reactions of the "temporarily able-bodied" toward those with disabilities, generally finding that the former hold negative attitudes about and avoid contact with the latter (Yuker, 1988). This avoidance may derive from society-wide stigmatizing attitudes, anxiety, embarrassment, not knowing what to say, or a host of other reasons created, in some measure, by lack of experience with the range of factors that can produce disability.

On the other hand, some authors have noted that positive inferences may be drawn by others about persons with disabilities on the assumption that there is something ennobling about living with a disability. As D. Dunn points out, this perspective is as flawed as its mirror image; it also focuses on the disability instead of the person with the condition and attributes some invariant quality to it instead of seeing "disability" as one aspect of the individual's being, interests, and abilities. Some interactions between persons with and without disabilities are affected by the "norm to be kind" (Hastorf, Northcraft, & Picciotto, 1979), another type of interaction shaped by social mores, not by the realities of the situation.

There is some evidence that individuals with disabilities can "defuse" tense social situations by casually offering an explanation of their disability or by being assertive (not aggressive) when asking for help (Hastorf, Wildfogel, & Cassman, 1979; Mills, Belgrave, & Boyer, 1984). M. Dunn (1987) described a social skills training program he developed to help prepare persons with recent-onset disability to handle common, potentially awkward social situations. Anticipatory role-playing ought to be considered for those expressing (understandable) apprehension about returning to the community in a newly disabled state.

Prevention

Many conditions for which rehabilitation is required are acquired; thus, preventive efforts can have a significant ultimate impact on the incidence of chronic illness and disability. For example, some public education programs have raised public awareness of stroke risk factors and initial symptoms (e.g., Reeves, Rafferty, Aranha, & Theisen, 2008), increasing the likelihood of earlier intervention and, consequently, reduced incidence and severity of disability from stroke. Wadley et al. (2007) identified five modifiable factors (hypertension, diabetes, smoking, lack of exercise, depressive symptoms), several of which appear treatable by behavioral methods familiar to psychologists. Those working in rehabilitation settings can provide a valuable service by helping patients to modify behaviors that put them at risk for (e.g.) stroke (Straus, Majumdar, & McAlister, 2002).

Given that the rehabilitation psychologist will typically encounter the rehabilitation patient only after onset of the disabling condition, *primary* prevention is not likely to be a major concern of the psychologist. However, prevention of *secondary* complications certainly falls within the psychologist's purview, encompassing, among other things, education about risk factors for recurrence and the importance of adherence to preventive treatment regimens. The technique of "motivational interviewing" (Miller & Rolnick, 2012)—a method of fostering intrinsic motivation to change maladaptive behaviors such as nonadherence and substance misuse—has been used with survivors of traumatic brain injury (Bombardier & Rimmele, 1999) and may well have considerable applicability to persons with other disabilities. Elliott, Kurylo, Chen, and Hicken (2002) found that those with new-onset spinal cord injury who had a history of alcohol abuse had an increased risk of pressure sores during the first 3 years after injury. These individuals would seem to be prime candidates for preventive intervention.

Outcomes Research

As noted earlier, measurement of outcome (and the associated goal of prediction of outcome) has long been emphasized in rehabilitation. An ever-present issue is deciding just what skills, interests, capacities, and so forth one should measure. These may well differ, depending on the case at hand; for one person mobility may be most salient, whereas another may be primarily concerned with return to work. Another relevant dimension is time since onset; measurement of short-term outcome (e.g., at discharge from rehabilitation) may address different domains (e.g., bathing, dressing) than longer term outcome where such matters as vocational status and quality of life may be paramount. The staggering breadth of outcome instruments is reflected in the recent compendium by Tate (2010), which reviews roughly 150 assessment measures. Although these instruments were specifically selected for use with those with brain injury, many are applicable to persons with other neurological disabilities.

Perhaps the most widely used functional outcome index is the Functional Independence Measure (FIM; Guide for the Uniform Data Set for Medical Rehabilitation, 1997), devised as a global outcome measure for persons with a wide variety of disabilities. Data have been reported on thousands of individuals, and the measure has good reliability and validity. However, the FIM is heavily weighted with motor items, and ceiling effects become common as time since onset increases, especially for certain populations such as those with acquired brain injury (e.g., Hall et al., 1996). Hall et al. (1996) even found ceiling effects for the FIM + FAM (Functional Assessment Measure), which includes 12 items specifically assessing cognitive skills such as reading, attention, and judgment not covered by the FIM. Interested readers might consult Tate's (2010) extensive overview of outcome measures grouped by the domain emphasized (e.g., sensorimotor functions, general and specific cognitive skills, quality of life, activities of daily living). Although as noted above, these were chosen for their applicability to brain injury, some have broader uses.

Lee, LoGallo, Banos, and Novack (2004) reported that neuropsychological outcome at 1 year after traumatic brain injury could be predicted by performance on brief cognitive screening measures. Sherer et al. (2002) showed the value of early neuropsychological testing in improving prediction of "productivity" in persons admitted to the Traumatic Brain Injury Model Systems facilities. Similar findings were reported by Boake et al. (2001). Hanks, Millis, and Ricker (2008) found that early cognitive screening results were associated with later need for supervision. Bowman (1996) concluded that testing after discharge contributed to predictions of success in returning to work, and Green et al. (2008) found testing at 5 months postinjury to be associated with "productivity" (e.g., paid employment, volunteer work, school, parenting) at 1 year for individuals with traumatic brain injury, whereas earlier (8 weeks postonset) testing revealed only a nonsignificant trend.

Diversity Issues

Rehabilitation psychology has a long history of sensitivity to the *au courant* concept of "diversity." In recent years, "disability" itself has come to be viewed as a diversity factor (Olkin, 2002), along with gender, ethnicity, cultural background, sexual orientation, spiritual preferences, and the like. There is an accumulating literature documenting the desirability of taking these factors into account in delivering clinical services. In their introduction to an issue of *Journal of Head Trauma Rehabilitation* devoted to cultural issues, Arango-Lasprilla and Niemeier (2007) summarized the findings of the contributing authors, noting cultural or racial disparities in prevalence of brain injury, rates of disability, employment outcomes, caregiver depression, and use of services.

Spiritual beliefs—not necessarily rooted in active practice of an organized religion (Waldron-Perrine, et al, 2011)—can affect the course of emotional response to disability, although not necessarily in a predictable fashion. Some deeply religious individuals with a new-onset disability may find emotional sustenance in their beliefs whereas others of similar faith may feel betrayed. Nonetheless, rehabilitation psychologists are increasingly aware of the need to explore spiritual values (Albright, Forchheimer, & Tate, 2010). Waldron-Perrine et al. (2011) found that survivors of traumatic brain injury who felt connected to a "higher power" had higher scores on measures of life satisfaction and functional abilities and a lower score on an index of emotional distress. Interestingly, it was the beliefs—not religious activity per se—that had predictive validity.

Substance Abuse and Disability

On a daily basis, rehabilitation psychologists encounter patients who owe their disability to misuse of drugs and/or alcohol. The estimated incidence of preinjury abuse or dependence ranges roughly between 15% and 66%, and studies of substance use at the time of injury have produced ranges of approximately one third to one half (Bombardier & Turner, 2010). Studies have found that the presence of preinjury problems with alcohol or drugs predicts several types of postinjury problems including the previously discussed higher incidence of pressure sores (Elliott et al., 2002) and depression (Dryden et al., 2005) in persons with spinal cord injury and increased risk of mortality in those with traumatic brain injury (Corrigan, 1995).

Concern about patients' drug and alcohol use does not abate with the end of inpatient rehabilitation. In many cases, postinjury use of alcohol and/or drugs is strictly contraindicated due to possible interaction with disability-related medications or concern about lowering inhibitions and placing the person at risk for further injury. For example, persons who reported receiving drug or alcohol treatment after spinal cord injury had an increased likelihood of requiring hospitalization for pressure sores (Krause, Vines, Farley, Sniezek, & Coker, 2001). Studies suggest that although substance use declines in the immediate aftermath of injury, it increases later on as the individual's mobility improves, bringing with it easier access to alcohol and drugs (Bombardier & Turner, 2010).

The emotional consequences of substance use–related injury can take varying forms. In some instances, patients feel tremendous guilt and self-blame for having indulged in behavior that has lifelong regrettable consequences for themselves and their families. Persons with strong religious beliefs may undergo a spiritual crisis. Others consider themselves victimized by random misfortune and do not see their substance use as a therapeutic issue. Given the potential implications of substance use and misuse, the competent rehabilitation psychologist should possess a reasonable familiarity with basic psychopharmacological concepts and practices.

Conclusion

The preceding review offers a broad but necessarily limited overview of some of the extant empirical support for certain practices of rehabilitation psychologists. With (a) increased survival rates for persons with disabling injuries and conditions, (b) an aging population that will increasingly need (and demand) rehabilitation services, and (c) an ever more financially strained health care system that increasingly places a premium on evidence-based treatments, there is a pressing need to continue to enlarge the scientific support for rehabilitation psychology services. Practitioners of rehabilitation psychology—with their broad-based training and skills and frequent placement in team treatment settings—are well suited to conduct ecologically relevant research on rehabilitation psychology topics specifically and to orchestrate multidisciplinary investigations involving other members of the rehabilitation enterprise.

ELEVEN

Supervision, Teaching, and Management

In addition to direct clinical care, supervision, teaching, and/or management can be important aspects of the work of some rehabilitation psychologists. Recognizing that a limited number of rehabilitation psychologists engage in these areas, the American Board of Rehabilitation Psychology has designated competence in them as complementary to the required competency areas. Nonetheless, some coverage is in order, given the increasing role they play in the specialty as it evolves.

Although these areas are distinct in several ways, they overlap significantly in others (e.g., typically the responsibility of more senior individuals, with accompanying power and authority differentials; somewhat removed from daily clinical practice; delivered to multiple subordinates or students). For the sake of brevity and (we hope) clarity, the terms *supervision* and *supervisor* are used, but readers should consider that *teaching/teacher, managing/manager,* or *administrating/administrator* could often be substituted. We do not intend to detail the various supervisory, teaching, and management roles, but rather to briefly address some of their commonalities. Interested readers are directed to the references for further discussion.

Evolution of Supervision Competency

There are many definitions of "supervision"; Bernard and Goodyear (1998) offer the following useful formulation that supervision is

> …an intervention provided by a more senior member of a profession to a more junior member or members of that same

profession. This relationship is evaluative, extends over time, and has the simultaneous purposes of enhancing the professional functioning of the more junior person(s), monitoring the quality of professional services offered to the client(s) she, he, or they see(s), and serving as a gatekeeper of those who are to enter the particular profession (p. 5).

The American Psychological Association (APA) "Ethical Principles of Psychologists and Code of Conduct" (2002, 2010a) contains only two provisions dealing with supervision:

> 7.06 Assessing Student and Supervisee Performance
> (a) In academic and supervisory relationships, psychologists establish a timely and specific process for providing feedback to students and supervisees. Information regarding the process is provided to the student at the beginning of supervision.
> (b) Psychologists evaluate students and supervisees on the basis of their actual performance on relevant and established program requirements.

Thus, supervisors must ensure that supervisees have a clear initial understanding of their responsibilities, how they will receive supervisory feedback, and the basis for performance ratings.

With the advent of competency-based education and training, supervision has come under increasing scrutiny in recent years. Bernard and Goodyear (2009) offer an overview of the various supervisory functions including monitoring services provided to clients, facilitating improvement in functional capabilities of less senior professionals, and tending to the "gateway" of the profession. Integrity, grounding in professional ethics, and understanding of—and tolerance for—diversity are key characteristics of supervisors (Falender & Shafranske, 2004).

Stoltenberg and Grus (2004) noted that supervision is an aspect of psychology practice for which there has historically been little formal training or standards; they also provide a history of the evolution of supervisory requirements. Most clinicians lack formal training and supervision in this area (Scott, Ingram, Vitanza, & Smith, 2000). Nonetheless, there seems to have been an implicit assumption that through one's own training, one came to understand psychological processes and concepts; hence, one could instruct and nurture budding psychologists. However, it is now understood that supervision is a distinct competency and requires a unique advanced set of skills and training.

Kaslow, Falender, and Grus (2012) list elements of competent supervision including observation, assisting the supervisee in self-assessment, provision of feedback and evaluation, and role-modeling, among others. The supervisor–supervisee relationship involves a balance of various roles and functions that at once satisfy the needs of the supervisee and tend to the responsibility of being a professional gatekeeper. Supervising effectively may be grounded in a transactional leadership style (e.g., providing objectives, directives, and goals) and/or a transformational leadership approach (e.g., encouraging creative thinking and innovation). With the increased trust and other positives associated with implementation of a transformational leadership style, Kaslow et al. (2012) anticipate that trainees will receive improved supervision, and the outcome will be more competent professionals and consumers who are better-served.

Some Inherent Issues

In all supervisory relationships, the highest ethical standards regarding interpersonal relationships must be upheld. Ladany and Lehrman-Waterman (1999) found that 51% of all supervisees reported witnessing at least one ethical violation by their supervisors. The violations were broad and ranged from conflicts of interest to sexual impropriety. Contracts between the supervisor and supervisee help to establish boundaries, spell out expectations, and foster adherence to deadlines and organizational requirements; sample contracts are available (Falender & Shafranske, 2004).

Open discussion at the outset of the relationship can help to establish and clarify the nature of the desired relationship and the expected behavior on both sides. Because internships are usually in partial fulfillment of requirements of an academic degree program and/or professional licensing, the demands of the degree granting institution, the jurisdictional authority for training, the requirements of the relevant professional body (usually the APA), and the expectations of the intern all must be given due consideration in the supervisory process.

Supervisors must strive to maintain empathy while not entering into overt or subtle emotional relationships that create irrelevant and/or counterproductive motivations and/or alternative methods of supervision.

Experience in the rehabilitation arena is frequently a differentiating factor that leads to an individual becoming a supervisor. Although skills and techniques may be taught, experience comes only with time, challenges, successes, and failures. The nuances of culture, politics, professionalism, and organizational management and the purpose and meaning of professional relationships are acquired through years of experience but such wisdom can be passed on within the scope of supervision, administration, and teaching.

Supervising and teaching prospective rehabilitation psychologists is doubtless one of the most important methods of ensuring the continuity of the profession and incorporating the latest knowledge, technology, and skills into daily clinical practice. Simply to have mastered a basic arsenal of information for practice does not equip one to teach or supervise. Regrettably, these areas receive minimal attention in most academic programs, leaving the practitioner at a loss when confronted with interns and residents who are there to learn (Johnson, DiLillo, & Garbin, 2010).

Perhaps one of the most salient features of a good supervisor is the ability to foster a keen sense of inquiry, motivation for lifelong learning, and willingness to move into new methods, technologies, and practice models while maintaining the strictest practice ethics and patient safety.

Modeling is paramount. Students (interns, residents, and others) perceive more than is intended to be transmitted and will imitate those who teach them. Arrogance, bigotry, and other negative attitudes will detract from anything that is verbally taught. Many conditions that present themselves in rehabilitation settings are emotionally taxing for the new practitioner. There are odors, mobility and mental dysfunctions, physical deformities, and other aversive experiences to be accepted and addressed. The way a supervisor approaches these situations automatically announces one's true empathy for and sincere interest in the patient, and one's competence for coping with these circumstances.

Supervising may be more a matter of modeling than didactic teaching. Although direct instruction is inevitable, as questions are posed for the supervisee to research and answer, cases are often *discussed* rather than *solved*. Good supervisors show *how* to learn, *what* to learn, and *the value* of learning. They do not threaten, but challenge. They *ask* more often than *answer,* and *mentor* as well as *monitor.*

Of particular importance are issues of diversity, individual differences, self-control, flexibility, the ability to think critically, tolerance, and maintaining an eagerness to learn and a willingness to accept supervision. Supervisors who are responsible for several levels of trainees (e.g., students, interns, and postdoctoral persons within the same program) must understand differing needs and make accommodations to meet them in creative ways, such as seminars, grand rounds, workshop formats, and additional one-on-one sessions.

The rehabilitation psychologist may be asked to supervise both other psychologists and nonpsychology professionals who confront psychological issues while practicing in rehabilitation settings. Frequently, occupational/recreational/physical therapists, social workers, and others within a rehabilitation team request supervision on aspects of their work as relates to a particular emotional, cognitive, or behavioral problem or other "psychological" domain.

The effective supervisor will introduce various models of supervision to help the supervisee understand differing clinical approaches and to reconfigure one's manner of thinking, method of presentation, and expected outcomes. It is vital that the supervisor promote growth in the trainee's capacity to conceptualize cases for grand rounds, team presentations, case conferences, report preparation, and potentially expert witness testimony. The supervisor may well be expected to teach the supervisee how to manage these various requirements.

Integrating and moving comfortably among multiple roles is important for both the supervisor and the supervisee. Both need to be able to provide critical but nonconfrontational feedback; hence, the establishment of trust is a key element in effective supervision. Both supervisee *and* supervisor need to participate in ongoing evaluation, and it is important that the supervisor be willing to entertain proper feedback from a supervisee in a nondefensive manner.

Supervisors must guard against emotional (or physical) complications with a supervisee. Both supervisor and supervisee may need to move beyond their "comfort level" and address the topics of transference and countertransference. It is of the utmost importance that unsuitable attitudes, actions, and professional indiscretions be addressed promptly. The actions and inactions of the supervisee are the responsibility of the supervisor as well. Failing to address such issues may reflect on the supervisor's competence, ethics, and reputation. Further, a fundamental aspect of the "contract" between supervisor and supervisee will have been breached, and patients potentially harmed. The supervisor's responsibility for both the supervisee and the supervisee's patients cannot be overstated.

At times, the supervisor may not be able to offer effective supervision to a particular individual due to differences in personality, prejudicial factors, or other reasons; these must be assessed fairly and addressed openly. When such occurs, referral to another supervisor is mandatory, with the referring supervisor addressing the issue with academic, organizational, or governing bodies as required.

There are critical differences between supervising psychology students and health service providers from other disciplines. The licensed individual presents requirements set forth by the state for both the supervisor and the supervisee. The nonpsychologist will usually come from some other behavioral or medical field but on occasion may represent the clergy, law, education, or other contributing party to a particular case. The principles of supervision do not change, but the specifics and focus undoubtedly will. In all cases, the code of conduct and specific organizational, educational, legal, and discipline-based requirements must be understood and met. In some cases, specified reporting to licensing boards is to be followed, and in other cases the supervisor is responsible to a graduate university program. It is important to recognize that supervision is not casual chatting or simply "going over a case" with a supervisee, but a crucial professional relationship with attendant expectations and requirements.

Supervision varies markedly according to the kind of program and institution. Supervisors in charge of a training program must be keenly aware of the guidelines set forth by the APA Division of Rehabilitation Psychology (Stiers et al., 2012) and by the American Board of Rehabilitation Psychology of the American Board of Professional Psychology.

Organizations often need assistance in understanding the funding, scheduling, staff requirements, trainee requirements, legal requirements, and many more details to carry out a responsible program. Further, the administration and staff of training institutions frequently are not sufficiently knowledgeable about rehabilitation psychology to understand the need for integration, team involvement, and staff privileges afforded to credentialed rehabilitation psychologists. Supervision in most educational and medical institutions results in more teaching and education than in direct one-on-one supervision. Developing good interdisciplinary professional relationships is an essential skill in being effective in program development and administration.

Certain sensitive issues may arise in the course of supervision. Among them are biases regarding religion, ethnicity, and political views; even the matter of quality of life with a disability may prove controversial. Although it is incumbent upon supervisors not to impose their views upon the supervisee, discussion of these issues may be encouraged so as to promote clarity of goals, purposes, and objectives in supervision. Maintaining neutrality may be desired but rarely successfully accomplished, and an understanding and respect for differing points of view is essential.

REFERENCES

Abrahamson, D. J., Steele, L. P., & Abrahamson, L. S. (2003). Practice, policy, and parity: The politics of persistence. *Professional Psychology: Research and Practice, 34,* 535–539.

Albright, K., Forchheimer, M., & Tate, D. (2010). Spirituality and rehabilitation. In R. Frank, M. Rosenthal, & B. Caplan (Eds.), *Handbook of rehabilitation psychology* (2nd ed., pp. 365–370). Washington, DC: American Psychological Association.

Alexander, T., & Wilz, G. (2010). Family caregivers: Gender differences in adjustment to stroke survivors' mental changes. *Rehabilitation Psychology, 55,* 159–169.

Allen, J., Litten, R., Fertig, J., & Babor, T. (1997). A review of research on the Alcohol Use Disorders Identification Test (AUDIT). *Alcoholism: Clinical and Experimental Research, 21,* 613–619.

American Bar Association and American Psychological Association. (2008). *Assessment of older adults with diminished capacity: A handbook for psychologists.* Washington, DC: Author.

American Board of Rehabilitation Psychology. (2010). *American Board of Rehabilitation Psychology examiner's manual.* Chapel Hill, NC: American Board of Professional Psychology.

American Board of Rehabilitation Psychology. (2011). Examination manual. Retrieved March 20, 2011, from http://www.abpp.org/files/page-specific/3361%20Rehab/15_ABRP_Candidate_Manual.pdf

American Psychological Association. (2002). Ethical principles of psychologists and code of conduct. *American Psychologist, 57,* 1060–1073.

American Psychological Association. (2003). Guidelines on multicultural education, training, research, practice and organizational change for psychologists. *American Psychologist, 58,* 377–402.

American Psychological Association. (2006, October). *APA Task Force on the Assessment of Competence in Professional Psychology: Final report.* Washington, DC: Author.

American Psychological Association. (2010a). 2010 Amendments to the 2002 "Ethical principles of psychologists and code of conduct." *American Psychologist, 65,* 493.

American Psychological Association. (2010b). HIPAA for psychologists. Retrieved October 28, 2010, from http://www.apapracticecentral.org/business/hipaa/index.aspx

Annon, J. (1974). *The behavioral treatment of sexual problems (Vol. 1): Brief therapy.* Honolulu, HI: Enabling Systems.

Arango-Lasprilla, J., & Niemeier, J. (2007). Cultural issues in the rehabilitation of TBI survivors: Recent research and new frontiers. *Journal of Head Trauma Rehabilitation, 22,* 73–74.

Artman, L. K., & Daniels, J. A. (2010). Disability and psychotherapy practice: Cultural competence and practical tips. *Professional Psychology: Research and Practice, 41,* 442–448.

Ashkenazi, G., Hagglund, K., Lee, A., Swaine, Z., & Frank. R. (2010). Health policy 101: Fundamental issues in health care reform. In R. Frank, M. Rosenthal, & B. Caplan (Eds.), *Handbook of rehabilitation psychology* (2nd ed., pp. 439–449). Washington, DC: American Psychological Association.

Backhaus, S., Ibarra, S., Klyce, D., Trexler, L., & Malec, J. (2010). Brain injury coping skills group: A preventative intervention for patients with brain injury and their caregivers. *Archives of Physical Medicine and Rehabilitation, 91,* 840–848.

Barnett, S., Heinemann, A., Libin, A., Houts, A., Gassaway, J., Gupta, S.,...Brossart, D. (2012). Small N designs for rehabilitation research. *Journal of Rehabilitation Research and Development, 49,* 175–186.

Barrett, A., Buxbaum, L., Coslett, H., Edwards, E., Heilman, K., Hillis, A.,...Robertson, I. (2006). Cognitive rehabilitation interventions for neglect and related disorders: Moving from bench to bedside in stroke patients. *Journal of Cognitive Neuroscience, 18,* 1223–1236.

Basford, J., Rohe, D., Barnes, C., & DePompolo, R. (2002). Substance abuse attitudes and policies in US rehabilitation training programs: A comparison of 1985 and 2000. *Archives of Physical Medicine and Rehabilitation, 83,* 517–522.

Behnke, S. H. (2005). On being an ethical psychologist. *Monitor on Psychology, 36,* 114–115.

Benedict, R., Fischer, J., Archibald, C., Arnett, P., Beatty, W., Bobholz, J.,...Munschauer, F. (2002). Minimal neuropsychological assessment of MS patients: A consensus approach. *The Clinical Neuropsychologist, 16,* 381–397.

Bent, R. (1992). The professional core competency areas. In R. Peterson, J. Holland, R. Bent, E. Davis-Russell, G. Edwall, K. Polite,...G. Stricker (Eds.), *The core curriculum in professional psychology* (pp. 77–81). Washington, DC: American Psychological Association.

Bent, R. J., & Cox, R. H. (1991). Intervention competency. In R. L. Peterson, R. J. Bent, J. D. McHolland, E. Davis-Russell, G. E. Edwall, K. Polite,...G. Stricker (Eds.), *The core curriculum in professional psychology* (pp. 97–102). Washington, DC: American Psychological Association.

Ben-Yishay, Y., Silver, S., Piasetsky, E., & Rattok, J. (1987). Relationship between employability and vocational outcome after intensive holistic cognitive rehabilitation. *Journal of Head Trauma Rehabilitation, 2,* 35–48.

Berg, A., Palomaki, H., Lonnqvist, J., Lehtihalmes, M., & Kaste, M. (2005). Depression among caregivers of stroke survivors. *Stroke, 36,* 639–643.

Bernard, J. M., & Goodyear, R. K. (1998). *Fundamentals of clinical supervision* (2nd ed.). Boston: Allyn and Bacon.

Bernard, J. M., & Goodyear, R. K. (2009). *Fundamentals of clinical supervision* (4th ed.). Upper Saddle River, NJ: Pearson Education.

Berninger, V., Gans, B., St. James, P., & Connors, T. (1988). Modified WAIS-R for patients with speech and/or hand dysfunction. *Archives of Physical Medicine and Rehabilitation, 69,* 250–255.

Berry, J., Elliott, T., & Rivera, P. (2007). Resilient, undercontrolled, and overcontrolled personality prototypes among persons with spinal cord injury. *Journal of Personality Assessment, 89,* 292–302.

Blonder, L., Langer, S., Pettigrew, L., & Garrity, T. (2007). The effects of stroke disability on spousal caregivers. *NeuroRehabilitation, 22,* 85–92.

Boake, C., Millis, S., High, W., Delmonico, R., Kreutzer, J., & Rosenthal, M. (2001). Using early neuropsychological testing to predict long-term productivity outcome from traumatic brain injury. *Archives of Physical Medicine and Rehabilitation, 82,* 761–768.

Bombardier, C., & Rimmele, C. (1998). Alcohol use and readiness to change after spinal cord injury. *Archives of Physical Medicine and Rehabilitation, 79,* 1110–1115.

Bombardier, C., & Rimmele, C. (1999). Motivational interviewing to prevent alcohol abuse after traumatic brain injury: A case series. *Rehabilitation Psychology, 44,* 52–67.

Bombardier, C., Rimmele, C., & Zintel, H. (2002). The magnitude and correlates of alcohol and drug use before traumatic brain injury. *Archives of Physical Medicine and Rehabilitation, 83,* 1765–1773.

Bombardier, C., Stroud, M., Esselman, P., & Rimmele, C. (2004). Do preinjury alcohol problems predict poorer rehabilitation progress in persons with spinal cord injury? *Archives of Physical Medicine and Rehabilitation, 85,* 1488–1492.

Bombardier, C., & Turner, A. (2010). Alcohol and other drug use in traumatic disability. In R. Frank, M. Rosenthal, & B. Caplan (Eds.), *Handbook of rehabilitation psychology* (2nd ed., pp. 241–258). Washington, DC: American Psychological Association.

Bourestom, N., & Howard, M. (1965). Personality characteristics of three disability groups. *Archives of Physical Medicine and Rehabilitation, 46,* 626–632.

Bowen, A., & Lincoln, N. (2007). Cognitive rehabilitation for spatial neglect following stroke. *Cochrane Database of Systematic Reviews, 2,* CD003586.

Bowman, M. (1996). Ecological validity of neuropsychological and other predictors following head injury. *The Clinical Neuropsychologist, 10,* 382–396

Braga, L., DePaz, A., & Ylvisaker, M. (2005). Direct clinician-delivered versus indirect family-supported rehabilitation of children with traumatic brain injury: A randomized controlled trial. *Brain Injury, 19,* 819–831.

Brenner, L. A., Vanderploeg, R. D., & Terrio, H. (2009). Assessment and diagnosis of mild traumatic brain injury, posttraumatic stress disorder, and other polytrauma conditions: Burden of adversity hypothesis. *Rehabilitation Psychology, 54*(3), 239–246.

Brown, L., Stern, R., Cahn-Weiner, D., Rogers, B., Messer, M., Lennon, M., et al. (2005). Driving Scenes test of the Neuropsychological Assessment Battery and on-road driving performance in aging and very mild dementia. *Archives of Clinical Neuropsychology, 20,* 209–215.

Brownsberger, M. G. (2004). Interview with Dr. Beatrice A. Wright. *Rehabilitation Psychology News, 31,* 8–9.

Brucker, B. (1984). Biofeedback in rehabilitation. In C. Golden (Ed.), *Current topics in rehabilitation psychology* (pp. 173–199). Orlando, FL: Grune and Stratton.

Bruyère, S. M., & O'Keefe, J. (Eds.). (1994). *Implications of the Americans with Disabilities Act for psychology.* New York, NY: Springer Publishing.

Bruyère, S. M., & Peterson, D. B. (2005). Introduction to the special section on the International Classification of Functioning, Disability and Health: Implications for rehabilitation psychology. *Rehabilitation Psychology, 50,* 103–104.

Buckelew, S., Baumstark, D., Frank, R., & Hewett, J. (1990). Adjustment following spinal cord injury. *Rehabilitation Psychology, 35,* 101–109.

Buckelew, S., Conway, R., Parker, J., Deuser, W., Jennings, J.,Witty, T., Hewett, J.,...Kay, D. (1998). Biofeedback/relaxation training and exercise interventions for fibromyalgia: A prospective trial. *Arthritis Care and Research, 11,* 196–209.

Burney, J. P., Celeste, B. L., Johnson, J. D., Klein, N. C., Nordal, K. C., & Portnoy, S. M. (2009). Mentoring professional psychologists: Programs for career development, advocacy, and diversity. *Professional Psychology: Research and Practice, 40,* 292–298.

Bush, S. (2000). Intermanual differences in performing a visuoconstructional task. *Archives of Physical Medicine and Rehabilitation, 81,* 1151–1152.

Bush, S. S. (Ed.). (2005). *A casebook of ethical challenges in clinical neuropsychology.* New York, NY: Psychology Press.

Butt, L., & Caplan, B. (2010). The rehabilitation team. In R. G. Frank, M. Rosenthal, & B. Caplan (Eds.), *Handbook of rehabilitation psychology* (2nd ed., pp. 451–457). Washington, DC: American Psychological Association.

Callahan, C. D. (2010). Rehabilitating the health care organization: Administering psychology's opportunity. In R. G. Frank, M. Rosenthal, & B. Caplan (Eds.), *Handbook of rehabilitation psychology* (2nd ed., pp. 459–466). Washington, DC: American Psychological Association.

Callahan, C. D., & Barisa, M. (2005). Statistical process control and rehabilitation outcome: The single subject design reconsidered. *Rehabilitation Psychology, 50,* 24–33.

Campbell, J. M. (2006). *Essentials of clinical supervision.* New York, NY: Wiley.

Caplan, B. (1982). Neuropsychology in rehabilitation: It's role in evaluation and intervention. *Archives of Physical Medicine & Rehabilitation, 63,* 362–366.

Caplan, B. (1988). Nonstandard neuropsychological assessment: An illustration. *Neuropsychology, 2,* 13–17.

Caplan, B. (1995). Choose your words! *Rehabilitation Psychology, 40,* 233–240.

Caplan, B. (2010). Rehabilitation psychology and neuropsychology with stroke survivors. In R. Frank, M. Rosenthal, & B. Caplan (Eds.), *Handbook of rehabilitation psychology* (2nd ed., pp. 63–94). Washington, DC: American Psychological Association.

Caplan, B., & Caffery, D. (1992). Fractionating block design: Development of a test of visual-spatial analysis. *Neuropsychology, 6,* 385–394.

Caplan, B., & Reidy, K. (1996). Staff-patient-family conflicts in rehabilitation: Sources and solutions. *Topics in Spinal Cord Injury, 2,* 21–33.

Caplan, B., & Shechter, J. (1987). Denial and depression in disabling illness. In B. Caplan (Ed.), *Rehabilitation psychology desk reference* (pp. 133–170). Rockville, MD: Aspen Publishers.

Caplan, B., & Shechter, J. (1991). Vocational capacity with cognitive impairment. In S. Scheer (Ed.), *Medical perspectives in vocational assessment of impaired workers* (pp. 149–172). Rockville, MD: Aspen Publishers.

Caplan, B., & Shechter, J. (1993). Reflections on the "depressed," "unrealistic," "inappropriate," "manipulative," "unmotivated," "noncompliant," "denying," "maladjusted," "regressed," etc. patient. *Archives of Physical Medicine and Rehabilitation, 74,* 1123–1124.

Caplan, B., & Shechter, J. (1995). The role of nonstandard neuropsychological assessment in rehabilitation: History, rationale and examples. In L. A. Cushman & M. J. Scherer (Eds.), *Psychological assessment in medical rehabilitation* (pp. 359–392). Washington, DC: American Psychological Association.

Caplan, B., & Shechter, J. (2005). Test accommodations in geriatric neuropsychology. In S. S. Bush & T. A. Martin (Eds.), *Geriatric neuropsychology: Practice essentials* (pp. 97–114). New York, NY: Psychology Press.

Caplan, G. (1995). Types of mental health consultation. *Journal of Educational and Psychological Consultation, 6,* 7–21.

Cardoso, E., Pruett, S., Chan, F., & Tansey, T. (2006). Substance abuse assessment and treatment: The current training and practice of APA Division 22 members. *Rehabilitation Psychology, 51,* 175–178.

Catalo, D., Chan, F., Wilson, L., Chiu, C-Y., & Muller, V. (2011). The buffering effect of resilience on depression among individuals with spinal cord injury: A structural equation model,. *Rehabilitation Psychology, 56,* 200–211.

Chaytor, N., & Schmitter-Edgecombe, M. (2003). The ecological validity of neuropsychological tests: A review of the literature on everyday cognitive skills. *Neuropsychology Review, 13,* 181–187.

Chevarley, F., Thierr, M., Gill, C. J., Ryerson, A. B., & Nosek, M. A. (2006). Health, preventive health care and health care access among women with disabilities in the 1994–1995 National Health Interview Survey. *Women's Health Issues, 16,* 297–312.

Chiaravalloti, N., & DeLuca, J. (2010). Cognition and multiple sclerosis: Assessment and treatment. In R. Frank, M. Rosenthal, & B. Caplan (Eds.), *Handbook of rehabilitation psychology* (2nd ed., pp. 133–144). Washington, DC: American Psychological Association.

Chronister, J., & Chan, F. (2006). A stress process model of caregiving for individuals with traumatic brain injury. *Rehabilitation Psychology, 51,* 190–201.

Chwalisz, K., & Chan, F. (Eds.). (2008). Research and methodological advances and issues in rehabilitation psychology (entire issue). *Rehabilitation Psychology, 53.*

Chwalisz, K., & Dollinger, S. (2010). Evidence-based practice with family caregivers. In R. Frank, M. Rosenthal, & B. Caplan (Eds.), *Handbook of rehabilitation psychology* (2nd ed., pp. 301–311). Washington, DC: American Psychological Association.

Cicerone, K., Dahlberg, C., Kalmar, K., Langenbahn, D., Malec, J., Bergquist, T., et al. (2000). Evidence-based cognitive rehabilitation: Recommendations for clinical practice. *Archives of Physical Medicine and Rehabilitation, 81,* 1596–1615.

Cicerone, K., Dahlberg, C., Malec, J., Langenbahn, D., Felicetti, T., Kneipp, S., et al. (2005). Evidence-based cognitive rehabilitation: Updated review of the literature from 1998 through 2004. *Archives of Physical Medicine and Rehabilitation, 85,* 943–950.

Cicerone, K., Langenbahn, D., Braden, C., Malec, J., Kalmar, K., Fraas, M., ... Ashman, T. (2011). Evidence-based cognitive rehabilitation: Updated review of the literature from 2003 through 2008. *Archives of Physical Medicine and Rehabilitation, 92,* 519–530.

Cicerone, K., Levin, H., Malec, J., Stuss, D., & Whyte, J. (2006). Cognitive rehabilitation interventions for executive function: Moving from bench to bedside in patients with traumatic brain injury. *Journal of Cognitive Neuroscience, 18,* 1212–1222.

Code, C. (2000). The problem with RCTs. *Royal College of Speech Language Therapists' Bulletin, March,* 14–15.

Cooney, N., Zweben, A., & Fleming, M. (1995). Screening for alcohol problems and at-risk drinking in health care settings. In R. Hester & W. Miller (Eds.), *Handbook of alcoholism treatment approaches: Effective alternatives* (pp. 45–60). Boston, MA: Allyn & Bacon.

Corrigan, J. (1995). Substance abuse as a mediating factor in outcome from traumatic brain injury. *Archives of Physical Medicine and Rehabilitation, 76,* 302–309.

Corrigan, J., Bogner, J., Lamb-Hart, G., Heinemann, A., & Moore, D. (2005). Increasing substance abuse treatment compliance for persons with traumatic brain injury. *Psychology of Addictive Behaviors, 19,* 131–139.

Costa, P., & McCrae, R. (1992). Four ways five factors are basic. *Personality and Individual Differences, 13,* 653–665.

Cox, D. R. (2010). Board certification in professional psychology: Promoting competency and consumer protection. *The Clinical Neuropsychologist, 24,* 493–505.

Cox, D. R., & Goldberg, A. L. (2010). Assessment of disability: Social security disability evaluation. In E. Mpofu & T. Oakland (Eds.), *Assessment in rehabilitation and health* (pp. 192–204). Upper Saddle River, NJ: Merrill.

Cox, D. R., Hess, D. W., Hibbard, M. R., Layman, D. E., & Stewart, R. K., Jr. (2010). Specialty practice in rehabilitation psychology. *Professional Psychology: Research and Practice, 41,* 82–88.

Cox, D. R., & Mahaffey, R. B. (1994). Clinical research programs and the iterative development process: The development of the IBM THINKabletm system. In B. T. McMahon & R. W. Evans (Eds.), *The shortest distance: The pursuit of independence for persons with acquired brain injury* (pp. 57–71). Winter Park, FL: PMD Publishers Group.

Cox, D. R., & Sanders, D. A. (2002). *Cut the CRAP and resolve your problems.* Sanford, FL: Diogenes Consortium Press.

Craig, A. (2012). Resilience in people with physical disabilities. In P. Kennedy (Ed.), *The Oxford handbook of rehabilitation psychology* (pp. 474–491). New York, NY: Oxford University Press.

Craig, A., Hancock, K., & Dickson, H. (1994). A longitudinal investigation into anxiety and depression in the first 2 years following a spinal cord injury. *Paraplegia, 32,* 675–679.

Cubic, B., & Gouvier, W. (1996). The ecological validity of perceptual tests. In R. Sbordone & C. Long (Eds.), *Ecological validity of neuropsychological testing* (pp. 203–224). Delray Beach, FL: GR Press/St. Lucie Press.

Davis, L., Sander, A., Struchen, M., Sherer, M., Nakase-Richardson, R., & Malec, J. (2009). Medical and psychosocial predictors of caregiver distress and perceived burden following traumatic brain injury. *Journal of Head Trauma Rehabilitation, 24,* 145–154.

Davis-Russell, E., Forbes, W. T., Bascuas, J., & Duran, E. (1991). Ethnic diversity and the core curriculum. In R. L. Peterson, R. J. Bent, J. D. McHolland, E. Davis-Russell, G. E. Edwall, K. Polite, ... G. Stricker (Eds.), *The core curriculum in professional psychology* (pp. 147–151). Washington, DC: American Psychological Association.

Dembo, T., Leviton, G., & Wright, B. A. (1956). Adjustment to misfortune: A problem of social psychological rehabilitation. *Artificial Limbs, 3,* 4–62.

Department of Veteran's Affairs. (1997). *Assessment of competency and capacity of the older adult: A practice guideline for psychologists.* Milwaukee, WI: National Center for Cost Containment (NTIS No. PB97-147904) (summarized in Baker, R., Lichtenberg, P., & Moye, J., *Professional Psychology: Research and Practice, 29,* 149–154).

deRoon-Cassini, T., Mancini, A., Rusch, M., & Bonanno, G. (2010). Psychopathology and resilience following traumatic injury: A latent growth mixture model analysis. *Rehabilitation Psychology, 55,* 1–11.

deRoon-Cassini, T., St. Aubin, E., Valvano, A., Hastings, J., & Horn, P. (2009). Psychological well-being after spinal cord injury: Perception of loss and meaning making. *Rehabilitation Psychology, 54,* 306–314.

Diller, L. (1990). Fostering the interdisciplinary team: Fostering research in a society in transition. *Archives of Physical Medicine and Rehabilitation, 71,* 275–278.

Dise-Lewis, J., Lewis, H., & Reichardt, C. (2009). BrainSTARS: Pilot data on a team-based intervention program for students who have acquired brain injury. *Journal of Head Trauma Rehabilitation, 24,* 166–177.

Doleys, D. (2000). Chronic pain. In R. Frank & T. Elliott (Eds.), *Handbook of rehabilitation psychology* (pp. 185–204). Washington, DC: American Psychological Association.

Doleys, D., & Doherty, D. (2000). Psychological/behavioral assessment. In P. Raj (Ed.), *Practical management of pain* (3rd ed., pp. 403–438). Philadelphia, PA: Mosby.

Dreer, L., Elliott, T., Shewchuck, R., Berry, J., & Rivera, P. (2007). Family caregivers of persons with spinal cord injury: Predicting caregivers at risk for depression. *Rehabilitation Psychology, 52,* 351–357.

Dryden, D., Saunders, L., Rowe, B., May, L., Yiannakoulias, N., & Svenson, L. (2005). Depression following traumatic spinal cord injury. *Neuroepidemiology, 25,* 55–61.

Dunn, D. (2010). The social psychology of disability. In R. Frank, M. Rosenthal, & B. Caplan (Eds.), *Handbook of rehabilitation psychology* (2nd ed., pp. 379–390). Washington, DC: American Psychological Association.

Dunn, M. (1987). Social skills and rehabilitation. In B. Caplan (Ed.), *Rehabilitation psychology desk reference* (pp. 345–364). Rockville, MD: Aspen Publishers.

Dunn, M., Van Horn, E., & Herman, S. (1976). *Social skills and the spinal cord injured patient.* (Videotape No. NAC004-179). Washington, DC: National Audio Visual Center.

Eberhardt, J. L. (2005). Imaging race. *American Psychologist, 60,* 181–190.

Ehde, D. (2010). Applications of positive psychology to rehabilitation psychology. In R. Frank, M. Rosenthal, & B. Caplan (Eds.), *Handbook of rehabilitation psychology* (2nd ed., pp. 417–424). Washington, DC: American Psychological Association.

Elliott, T., & Frank, R. (1996). Depression following spinal cord injury. *Archives of Physical Medicine and Rehabilitation, 77,* 816–823.

Elliott, T. R., & Gramling, S. E. (1990). Psychologists and rehabilitation: New roles and old training models. *American Psychologist, 45,* 762–765.

Elliott, T., Herrick, S., Patti, A., Witty, T., Godshall, F., & Spruell, M. (1991). Assertiveness, social support, and psychological adjustment of persons with spinal cord injury. *Behaviour Research and Therapy, 29,* 485–493.

Elliott, T., Kurylo, M., Chen, Y., & Hicken, B. (2002). Alcohol history and adjustment following spinal cord injury. *Rehabilitation Psychology, 47,* 278–290.

Elliott, T., & Umlauf, R. (1995). Measurement of personality and psychopathology following acquire physical disability. In L. Cushman & M. Scherer (Eds.), *Psychological assessment in medical rehabilitation* (pp. 325–358). Washington, DC: American Psychological Association.

Elliott, T., Witty, T., Herrick, S., & Hoffman, J. (1991). Negotiating reality after physical loss: Hope, depression, and disability. *Journal of Personality and Social Psychology, 61,* 608–613.

Enders, C. (2011). Analyzing longitudinal data with missing values. *Rehabilitation Psychology, 56,* 2672–2688.

Engel, G. L. (1977). The need for a new medical model: A challenge for biomedicine. *Science, 196,* 129–136.

Epstein, N. B., Baldwin, L. M., & Bishop, D. S. (1983). The McMaster Family Assessment Device. *Journal of Marital and Family Therapy, 9,* 171–180.

Eslinger, P. (2002). *Neuropsychological interventions: Clinical research and practice.* New York, NY: Guilford Press.

Eskes, G., & Barrett, A. (2009).Neuropsychological rehabilitation. In J. Festa & R. Lazar (Eds.). *Neurovascular neuropsychology* (pp. 281–305). New York, NY: Springer.

Ewing, J. (1984). Detecting alcoholism: The CAGE questionnaire. *Journal of the American Medical Association, 252,* 1905–1907.

Falender, C. A., & Shafranske, E. M. (2004). *Clinical supervision: A competency-based approach.* Washington, DC: American Psychological Association.

Fields, A. J. (2010). Multicultural research and practice: Theoretical issues and maximizing cultural exchange. *Professional Psychology: Research and Practice, 41,* 196–201.

Flanagan, R., & Miller, J. A. (2010). *Specialty competencies in school psychology.* New York, NY: Oxford University Press.

Fordyce, W. E. (1964). Personality characteristics in men with spinal cord injury as related to manner of onset of disability. *Archives of Physical Medicine and Rehabilitation, 45,* 321–325.

Fordyce, W. E. (1976). *Behavioral methods for chronic pain and illness.* St. Louis, MO: Mosby.

Fordyce, W. E. (1982). Psychological assessment and management in rehabilitation. In F. Kottke, G. Stillwell, & J. Lehmann (Eds.), *Krusen's handbook of physical medicine and rehabilitation* (pp. 124–150). Philadelphia, PA: W. B. Saunders.

Frank, R. G., Gluck, J. P., & Beckelew, S. P. (1990). Rehabilitation: Psychology's greatest opportunity? *American Psychologist, 45,* 757–761.

Frankl, V. E. (2006). *Man's search for meaning.* Boston, MA: Beacon.

Fraser, R., & Johnson, K. (2010). Vocational rehabilitation. In R. G. Frank, M. Rosenthal, & B. Caplan (Eds.), *Handbook of rehabilitation psychology* (2nd ed., pp. 357–363). Washington, DC: American Psychological Association.

Frassinetti, F., Angeli, V., Meneghello, F., Avanzi, S., & Ladavas, E. (2002). Long-lasting amelioration of visuospatial neglect by prism adaptation. *Brain, 125,* 608–623.

Freeman, K., & Lim, M. (2010). Single subject research. In J. Thomas & M. Hersen (Eds.), *Handbook of clinical psychology competencies* (pp. 397–424). New York, NY: Springer.

Frew, J. (2010). Consultation. In J. C. Thomas & M. Hersen (Eds.), *Handbook of clinical psychology competencies* (pp. 549–572). New York, NY: Springer.

Gallaher, C., & Hough, S. (2001). Ethnicity and age issues: Attitudes affecting rehabilitation of individuals with spinal cord injury. *Rehabilitation Psychology, 46,* 312–321.

Gans, J. (1987). Facilitating staff-patient interaction in rehabilitation. In B. Caplan (Ed.), *Rehabilitation psychology desk reference* (pp. 185–218). Rockville, MD: Aspen Publishers.

Garrett, J., & Levine, E. (1961). *Psychological practices with the physically disabled.* New York, NY: Columbia University Press.

Gass, C. (1992). MMPI-2 interpretation of patients with cerebrovascular disease: A correction factor. *Archives of Clinical Neuropsychology, 7,* 17–27.

Gaugler, J. (2010). The longitudinal ramifications of stroke caregiving: A systematic review. *Rehabilitation Psychology, 55,* 108–125.

Geertz, C. (1973). *Interpretation of cultures.* New York, NY: Basic Books.

Gialanella, B., & Mattioli, F. (1992). Anosognosia and extrapersonal neglect as predictors of functional recovery following right hemisphere stroke. *Neuropsychological Rehabilitation, 2,* 169–178.

Gillen, G. (2005). Positive consequences of surviving a stroke. *American Journal of Occupational Therapy, 59,* 346–350.

Glueckauf, R. L. (2000). Doctoral education in rehabilitation and health care psychology: Principles and strategies for unifying subspecialty training. In R. G. Frank & T. Elliot (Eds.), *Handbook of rehabilitation psychology* (pp. 615–627). Washington, DC: American Psychological Association.

Gold, S., & De Piano, F. (1992). Assessment competency. In R. Peterson, J. Holland, R. Bent, E. Davis-Russell, G. Edwall, K. Polite,...G. Stricker (Eds.), *The core curriculum in professional psychology* (pp. 89–95). Washington, DC: American Psychological Association.

Goldstein, K. (1942). *After effects of brain injuries in war.* New York : Grune & Stratton.

Graham, J. M., & Kim, Y. H. (2011). Predictors of doctoral student success in professional psychology: Characteristics of students, programs, and universities. *Journal of Clinical Psychology, 67,* 340–354.

Grant, J., Elliott, T., Giger, J., & Bartolucci, A. (2001). Social problem-solving abilities, social support, and adjustment among family caregivers of individuals with a stroke. *Rehabilitation Psychology, 46,* 44–57.

Green, B., Colella, R., Hebert, D., Bayley, M., Kang, H., Till, C., & Monette, G. (2008). Prediction of return to productivity after severe traumatic brain injury: Investigations of optimal neuropsychological tests and timing of assessment. *Archives of Physical Medicine and Rehabilitation, 89*(12 Suppl. 2), S51–S60.

Griffith, E., & Lemberg, S. (1993). *Sexuality and the person with traumatic brain injury: A guide for families.* Philadelphia, PA: F. A. Davis.

Grober, S., Hibbard, M., Gordon, W., Stein, P., & Freeman, A. (1993). The psychotherapeutic treatment of post-stroke depression with cognitive behavioral therapy. In W. A. Gordon (Ed.), *Advances in stroke rehabilitation* (pp. 215–241). Andover, MA: Andover Medical Publishers.

Guide for the Uniform Data Set for Medical Rehabilitation (including the FIM instrument; Version 5.1) (1997). Buffalo, NY: State University of New York at Buffalo.

Guilmette, T., Hagan, L., & Giuliano, A. (2008). Assigning qualitative descriptors to test scores in neuropsychology: Forensic implications. *The Clinical Neuropsychologist, 22,* 122–139.

Gusman, F. D., Stewart, J., Young, B. H., Riney, S. J., Abueg, F. R., & Blake, D. D. (1996). A multicultural developmental approach for treating trauma. In A. J. Marsella, M. J. Friedman, J. Matthew, E. T. Gerrity, & R. M. Scurfield (Eds.), *Ethnocultural aspects of posttraumatic stress disorder: Issues, research, and clinical applications* (pp. 439–457). Washington, DC: American Psychological Association.

Hackett, M., & Anderson, C. (2005). Predictors of depression after stroke: A systematic review of observational studies. *Stroke, 36,* 2296–2301.

Hackett, M., Anderson, C., & House, A. (2005). Management of depression after stroke: A systematic review of pharmacologic therapies. *Stroke, 36,* 1092.

Hackett, M., Anderson, C., House, A., & Halteh, C. (2009). Interventions for prevention of depression after stroke. *Stroke, 40,* e485–e486.

Hackett, M., Anderson, C., House, A., & Xia, J. (2009). Interventions for treating depression after stroke. *Stroke, 40,* e487–e488.

Hall, K., Mann, N., High, W., Wright, J., Kreutzer, J., & Wood, D. (1996). Functional measures after traumatic brain injury: Ceiling effects of the FIM, FIM+FAM, DRS, and CIQ. *Journal of Head Trauma Rehabilitation, 11,* 27–39.

Hall, P., Marshall, J., Mercado, A., & Tkachuk, G. (2011). Changes in coping style and treatment outcome following motor vehicle accident. *Rehabilitation Psychology, 56,* 43–51.

Hanks, R., Millis, S., & Ricker, J. (2008). The predictive value of a brief neuropsychologic battery for persons with traumatic brain injury. *Archives of Physical Medicine and Rehabilitation, 89,* 950–957.

Hanoch, L., & Siller, J., (2004). Psychodynamic therapy. In F. Chan, N. Berven, & K. Thomas (Eds.), *Counseling Theories and Techniques for Rehabilitation Health Professionals.* (pp. 20–52). New York, NY: Springer.

Hanson, S., & Kerkhoff, T. (2007). Ethical decision-making in rehabilitation: Considerations of Latino cultural factors. *Rehabilitation Psychology, 52*(4), 409–420.

Hanson, S. L., & Kerkhoff, T. R. (2010). Ethics. In R. G. Frank, M. Rosenthal, & B. Caplan (Eds.), *Handbook of rehabilitation psychology* (2nd ed., pp. 427–437). Washington, DC: American Psychological Association.

Hart, T. (2009). Treatment definition in complex rehabilitation interventions. *Neuropsychological Rehabilitation, 19,* 824–940.

Hart, T. (2010). Cognitive rehabilitation. In R. G. Frank, M. Rosenthal, & B. Caplan (Eds.), *Handbook of rehabilitation psychology* (2nd ed., pp. 285–300). Washington, DC: American Psychological Association.

Hart, T., Fann, J., & Novack, T. (2008). The dilemma of the control condition in experience-based cognitive and behavioral treatment research. *Neuropsychological Rehabilitation, 18,* 1–21.

Hart, T., Sherer, M., Temkin, N., Whyte, J., Dikmen, S., Heinemann, A., & Bell, K. (2010). Participant-proxy agreement on objective and subjective aspects of societal participation following traumatic brain injury. *Journal of Head Trauma Rehabilitation, 21,* 339–348.

Hart, T., Vaccaro, M., Hays, C., & Mauiro, R. (2012). Anger self-management training for people with traumatic brain injury: A preliminary investigation. *Journal of Head Trauma Rehabilitation, 27,* 113–122.

Hartke, R., Heinemann, A., King, R., & Semik, P. (2006). Accidents in caregivers of persons surviving stroke and their relation to caregiver stress. *Rehabilitation Psychology, 51,* 150–156.

Hastorf, A., Northcraft, J., & Piccioto, S. (1979). Helping the handicapped: How realistic is the performance feedback received by the physically handicapped? *Journal of Personality and Social Psychology, 5,* 373–376.

Hastorf, A., Wildfogel, J., & Cassman, T. (1979). Acknowledgement of handicap as a tactic in social interaction. *Journal of Personality and Social Psychology, 37,* 1790–1797.

Hayes, S., Strosahl, K., Wilson, K., Bisset, R., Pistorello, J., Toarmino, D., et al. (2004). Measuring experiential avoidance: A preliminary test of a working model. *The Psychological Record, 54,* 553–578.

Heaton, R., & Pendleton, M. (1981). Use of neuropsychological tests to predict adult patients' everyday functioning. *Journal of Consulting and Clinical Psychology, 49,* 807–821.

Heinemann, A., & Mallinson, T. (2010). Functional status and quality of life measures. In R. Frank, M. Rosenthal, & B. Caplan (Eds.), *Handbook of rehabilitation psychology* (2nd ed., pp. 147–164). Washington, DC: American Psychological Association.

Heinrich, R., Tate, D., & Buckelew, S. (1994). Brief symptom inventory norms for spinal cord injury. *Rehabilitation Psychology, 35,* 217–228.

Hibbard, M., & Cox, D. (2010). Competencies of a rehabilitation psychologist. In R. G. Frank, B. Caplan, & M. Rosenthal (Eds.), *Handbook of rehabilitation psychology* (2nd ed., pp. 467–475). Washington, DC: American Psychological Association.

Hibbard, M. R., Layman, D. E., & Stewart, R. K., Jr. (2010). The neurorehabilitation psychologist. In E. R. Arzubi & E. Mambrino (Eds.), *A guide to neuropsychological testing for health care professionals* (pp. 369–394). New York, NY: Springer Publishing.

Hill-Briggs, F., Kirk, J., & Wegener, S. (2005). Geriatric pain and neuropsychological assessment. In S. Bush & T. Martin (Eds.), *Geriatric neuropsychology: Practice essentials* (pp. 385–400). New York, NY: Psychology Press.

Hollick, C., Radnitz, C., Silverman, J., Tirch, D., Birstein, S., & Bauman, W. (2001). Does spinal cord injury affect personality? A study of monozygotic twins. *Rehabilitation Psychology, 46,* 58–67.

Homaifar, B. Y. (2007). Interview with Nancy Crewe, Ph.D. *Rehabilitation Psychology News, Win, 34,* 12–13.

Horvath, A. O., & Bedi, R. P. (2002). The alliance. In J. C. Norcross (Ed.), *Psychotherapy relationships that work: Therapist contributions and responsiveness to patients* (pp. 89–108). New York, NY: Oxford University Press.

Hoskin, K., Jackson, H., & Crowe, S. (2005). Money management after acquired brain dysfunction: The validity of neuropsychological assessment. *Rehabilitation Psychology, 50,* 355–365.

Hughes, R., Robinson-Whelan, S., Taylor, H., Swedlund, N., & Nosek, M. (2004). Enhancing self-esteem in women with physical disabilities. *Rehabilitation Psychology, 49,* 295–302.

Ince, L. (1976). *Behavior modification in rehabilitation settings.* Springfield, IL: Charles Thomas.

Jackson, D. (2010). Reporting results of latent growth modeling and multilevel modeling analyses: Some recommendations for rehabilitation psychology. *Rehabilitation Psychology, 55,* 272–285.

Jacobs, H. E. (1993). *Behavior analysis guidelines and brain injury rehabilitation: People, principles and programs.* Gaithersburg, MD: Aspen Publishing Company.

Jacobson, N., Follette, R., & Revenstorff, D. (1984). Psychotherapy outcome research: Methods for reporting variability and evaluating clinical significance. *Behavior Therapy, 15,* 336–352.

Jensen, M., & Karoly, P. (2001). Self-report scales and procedures for assessing pain in adults. In D. Turk & R. Melzack (Eds.), *Handbook of pain assessment* (pp. 15–34). New York, NY: Guilford Press.

Jensen, M., & Karoly, P. (2007). *Survey of pain attitudes*. Bloomington, MN: Pearson Assessment.

Johnson, B., DiLillo, D., & Garbin, C. (2010). Teaching. In J. C. Thomas & M. Hersen (Eds.), *Handbook of clinical psychology competencies* (pp. 573–608). New York, NY: Springer.

Johnson, E. (2007). Psychologically healthy workplaces: A focus on rehabilitation facilities. *Rehabilitation Psychology News, 35*, 13.

Johnson-Greene, D., & Touradji, P. (2010). Assessment of personality and psychopathology. In R. Frank, M. Rosenthal, & B. Caplan (Eds.), *Handbook of rehabilitation psychology* (2nd ed., pp. 195–212). Washington, DC: American Psychological Association.

Johnstone, B., & Stonington, H. (Eds.). (2009). *Rehabilitation of neuropsychological disorders*. New York, NY: Psychology Press.

Jorge, R., Robinson, R., Arndt, S., & Starkstein, S. (2003). Mortality and poststroke depression: A placebo-controlled trial of antidepressants. *American Journal of Psychiatry, 160*, 1823–1829.

Judd, T., & Fordyce, D. (1996). Personality tests. In R. Sbordone & C. Long (Eds.), *Ecological validity of neuropsychological testing* (pp. 315–355). Delray Beach, FL: GR Press/St. Lucie Press.

Kahan, J., Mitchell, J., Kemp, B., & Adkins, R. (2006). The results of a 6-month treatment for depression on symptoms, life satisfaction, and community activities among individuals aging with a disability. *Rehabilitation Psychology, 51*, 13–22.

Kaslow, N. J., Falender, C. A., & Grus, C. L. (2012). Valuing and practicing competency-based supervision: A transformational leadership perspective. *Training and Education in Professional Psychology, 6*, 47–54.

Kaslow, N. J., Rubin, N. J., Bebeau, M. J., Leigh, I. W., Lichtenberg, J. W., Nelson, P. D., ... & Smith, I. L. (2007). Guiding principles and recommendations for the assessment of competence. *Professional Psychology Research and Practice, 38*(5), 441–451.

Katz, N., Ring, H., Naveh, Y., Kizony, R., Feintuch, U., & Weiss, P. (2005). Interactive virtual environment training for safe street crossing of right hemisphere stroke patients with unilateral spatial neglect. *Disability and Rehabilitation, 27*, 1235–1243.

Keany, K., & Glueckauf, R. (1993). Disability and value change: An overview and reanalysis of acceptance of loss theory. *Rehabilitation Psychology, 38*, 199–210.

Kennedy, P., Duff, J., Evans, M., & Beedie, A. (2003). Coping effectiveness training reduces depression and anxiety following traumatic spinal cord injuries. *Journal of Clinical Psychology, 42*, 41–52.

Kennedy, P., & Rogers, B. (2000). Anxiety and depression after spinal cord injury: A longitudinal analysis. *Archives of Physical Medicine and Rehabilitation, 81*, 932–937.

Kennedy, P. (Ed.). (2012). *The Oxford handbook of rehabilitation psychology*. New York, NY: Oxford University Press.

Kerns, R., Turk, D., & Rudy, T. (1995). The West Have-Yale multidimensional pain inventory. *Pain, 23*, 245–256.

Kirsch, N., & Scherer, M. (2010). Assistive technology for cognition and behavior. In R. Frank, M. Rosenthal, & B. Caplan (Eds.), *Handbook of rehabilitation psychology* (2nd ed., pp. 273–284). Washington, DC: American Psychological Association.

Kirsch, N., Shenton, M., Spirl, E., Simpson, R., LoPresti, E., & Schreckenghost, D. (2004). Modifying verbose speech after traumatic brain injury with an assistive technology system for coordinated behavior change cueing and monitoring. *Journal of Head Trauma Rehabilitation, 19,* 366–377.

Kortte, K., Gilbert, M., Gorman, P., & Wegener, S. (2010). Positive psychological variables in the prediction of life satisfaction after spinal cord injury. *Rehabilitation Psychology, 55,* 40–47.

Kortte, K., Stevenson, J., Hosey, M., & Wegener, S. (2012). Hope predicts positive functional outcomes in acute rehabilitation populations. *Rehabilitation Psychology, 57,* 248–255.

Kortte, K., Veiel, L., Batten, S., & Wegener, S. (2009). Measuring avoidance in medical rehabilitation. *Rehabilitation Psychology, 54,* 91–98.

Kortte, K., Gilbert, M., Gorman, P., & Wegener, S. (2010). Positive psychological variables in the prediction of life satisfaction after spinal cord injury. *Rehabilitation Psychology, 55,* 40–47.

Krause, J., Vines, C., Farley, T., Sniezek, J., & Coker, J. (2001). An exploratory study of pressure ulcers after spinal cord injury: Relationship to protective behaviors and risk factors. *Archives of Physical Medicine and Rehabilitation, 82,* 107–113.

Kreutzer, J., Marwitz, J., & Witol, A. (1996). Interrelationships between crime, substance abuse, and aggressive behavior among persons with traumatic brain injury. *Brain Injury, 9,* 757–768.

Kubler-Ross, E. (1969). *On death and dying.* New York, NY: Collier-MacMillan.

Kurtz, J., Putnam, S., & Stone, C. (1998). Stability of normal personality traits after traumatic brain injury. *Journal of Head Trauma Rehabilitation, 13,* 1–14.

La Roche, M., & Christopher, M. S. (2010). Cultural diversity. In J. C. Thomas & M. Hersen (Eds.), *Handbook of clinical psychology competencies* (pp. 95–122). New York, NY: Springer.

Ladany, N., & Lehrman-Waterman, D. (1999). The content and frequency of supervisor self-disclosures and their relationship to supervisor style and the supervisory working alliance. *Counselor Education and Supervision, 38,* 143–160.

Lakes, K., Lopez, S. R., & Garro, L. C. (2006). Cultural competence and psychotherapy: Applying anthropologically informed conceptions of culture. *Psychotherapy: Theory, Research, Practice, & Training, 43,* 380–396.

Larson, E., Kirschner, K., Bode, R., Heinemann, A., Clorfene, J., & Goodman, R. (2003). Brief cognitive assessment and prediction of functional outcome in stroke. *Topics in Stroke Rehabilitation, 9,* 10–21.

Larson, P. C., & Sachs, P. R. (2000). A history of Division 22 (Rehabilitation Psychology). In D. A. Dewsbury (Ed.), *Unification through division: Histories of the divisions of the American Psychological Association* (Vol. V, pp. 33–58). Washington, DC: American Psychological Association.

Lauritzen, L., Bjerg Bendsen, B., Vilmar, T., Bjerg Bendsen, E., Lunde, M., & Bech, P. (1994). Post stroke depression: Combined treatment with imipramine or desipramine and mianserin. *Psychopharmacology, 114,* 119–122.

Lazarus, R., & Folkman, S. (1984). *Stress, appraisal, and coping.* New York, NY: Springer.

Leahy, M. (1995). Assessment of vocational interests and aptitudes in rehabilitation settings. In L. Cushman & M. Scherer (Eds.), *Psychological assessment in medical rehabilitation* (pp. 299–324). Washington, DC: American Psychological Association.

Leibowitz, R., & Stanton, A. (2007). Sexuality after spinal cord injury: A conceptual model based on women's narratives. Rehabilitation Psychology, 52, 44–55.

Lee, D., LoGalbo, A., Banos, J., & Novack, T. (2004). Prediction of cognitive abilities 1 year following traumatic brain injury from rehabilitation screening. *Rehabilitation Psychology, 49,* 167–171.

Lengenfelder, J., Chiaravalloti, N., & DeLuca, J. (2007). The efficacy of the generation effect in improving new learning in persons with traumatic brain injury. *Rehabilitation Psychology, 52,* 290–296.

Lenze, E., Munin, M., Quear, T., Dewe, M., Rogers, J., Begley, A., et al. (2004). Significance of poor patient participation in physical and occupational therapy for functional outcome and length of stay. *Archives of Physical Medicine and Rehabilitation, 85,* 1599–1601.

Levenkron, J. (1987). Behavior modification in rehabilitation: Principles and clinical strategies. In B. Caplan (Ed.), *Rehabilitation psychology desk reference* (pp. 383–410). Rockville, MD: Aspen Publishers.

Lewis, B. L., Hatcher, R. L., & Pate, W. E. (2005). The Practicum Experience: A survey of practicum site coordinators. *Professional Psychology: Research and Practice, 36,* 291–298.

Lichtenberg, P., & Schneider, B. (2010). Psychological assessment and practice in geriatric rehabilitation. In R. G. Frank, B. Caplan, & M. Rosenthal (Eds.), *Handbook of rehabilitation psychology* (2nd ed., pp. 95–106). Washington, DC: American Psychological Association.

Lincoln, N., & Flannaghan, T. (2003). Cognitive behavioral psychotherapy for depression following stroke: A randomized controlled trial. *Stroke, 34,* 111–115.

Loeb, P. (2003). *The independent living scales.* San Antonio, TX: Pearson Assessment.

Lollar, D. (2008). Rehabilitation psychology and public health: Commonalities, barriers, and bridges. *Rehabilitation Psychology, 53,* 122–127.

Lomay, V., & Hinkebein, J. (2006). Cultural considerations when providing rehabilitation services to American Indians. *Rehabilitation Psychology, 51,* 36–42.

Lopez, W. L. (2005). Interview with Dr. Wilbert E. Fordyce. *Rehabilitation Psychology News, 33,* 6.

LoSasso, G., Rapport, L., Axelrod, B., & Reeder, K. (1998). Intermanual and alternate-form equivalence in the Trail Making Test. *Journal of Clinical and Experimental Neuropsychology, 20,* 107–110.

Lubin, B., Larsen, R., Matarazzo, J., & Seever, M. (1986). Selected characteristics of psychologists and psychological assessment in five settings: 1959–1982. *Professional Psychology, 17,* 155–157.

Lubin, B., & Lubin, A. (1972). Patterns of psychological services in the US: 1959–1969. *Professional Psychology, 3,* 63–65.

Luginbuehl, M. (2008). Assessment of sleep problems in a school setting or private practice. In A. Ivanenko (Ed.), *Sleep and Psychiatric Disorders in Children and Adolescents* (pp. 109–138). New York, NY: Informa Healthcare.

Luria, A. R. (1963). *Restoration of function after brain injury.* New York: Pergamon Press.

Lynch, E.W., & Hanson, M. J. (Eds.) (2004). *Developing cross cultural competence: A guide for working with Children and their families* (3d ed.). Baltimore: Paul H. Brookes Publishing Co.

Malec, J., & Moessner, A. (2000). Self-awareness, distress, and rehabilitation outcome. *Rehabilitation Psychology, 45,* 227–241.

Marcotte, T., & Grant, I. (Eds.). (2010). *Neuropsychology of everyday functioning*. New York, NY: Guilford Press.

Marson, D., Dreer, L., Krzywanski, S., Huthwaite, J., DeVivo, M., & Novack, T. (2005). Impairment and partial recovery of medical decision-making capacity in traumatic brain injury. *Archives of Physical Medicine and Rehabilitation, 86*, 889–895.

Marson, D., Sawrie, S., Snyder, S., McInturff, B., Stalvery, T., Boothe, A., et al. (2000). Assessing financial capacity in patients with Alzheimer's disease: A conceptual model and prototype instrument. *Archives of Neurology, 57*, 877–884.

McAweeney, M., & Crewe, N. (2000). Evaluating outcomes research: Statistical concerns and clinical relevance. In R. Frank & T. Elliott (Eds.), *Handbook of rehabilitation psychology* (pp. 311–326). Washington, DC: American Psychological Association.

McGrath, J., & Linley, P. (2006). Posttraumatic growth in acquired brain injury: A preliminary small scale study. *Brain Injury, 20*, 767–773.

McHolland, J., Peterson, D. R., & Brown, S. W. (1987). Assessing skills in professional psychology: A triadic strategy for developing methods. In E. F. Bourg, R. J. Bent, J. E. Callan, N. F. Jones, J. McHolland, & G. Stricker (Eds.), *Standards and evaluation in the education and training of professional psychologists: Knowledge, attitudes and skills* (pp. 105–128). Norman, OK: Transcript Press.

McMillen, J., & Cook, C. (2003). The positive by-products of spinal cord injury and their correlates. *Rehabilitation Psychology, 48*, 77–85.

McPherson, C., & Addington-Hall, J. (2003). Judging the quality of care at the end of life: Can proxies provide reliable information? *Social Science and Medicine, 56*, 95–109.

Mehta, S., Orenczuk, S., Hansen, K., Aubut, J., Hitzig, S., Legassic, M., & Teasell, R. (2011). An evidence-based review of the effectiveness of cognitive behavioral therapy for psychosocial issues post-spinal cord injury. *Rehabilitation Psychology, 56*, 15–25.

Melzack, R. (2005). The McGill pain questionnaire: From description to measurement. *Anesthesiology, 103*, 199–202.

Meyerink, L., Reitan, R., & Selz, M. (1988). The validity of the MMPI in multiple sclerosis. *Journal of Clinical Psychology, 44*, 764–769.

Meyerson, L. (1957). Special disabilities. *Annual Review of Psychology, 8*, 437–457.

Meyerson, L. (1963). Perspectives: The life and times of the Division on Psychological Aspects of Disability—An intellectual history. *Division 22 Bulletin, 10*(3), 40–46. APA Division 22 Rehabilitation Psychology.

Miller, L., & Donders, J. (2003). Prediction of educational outcome after traumatic brain injury. *Rehabilitation Psychology, 48*, 237–241.

Miller, W., & Rollnick, S. (2012). *Motivational interviewing: Preparing people to change addictive behaviors* (3rd ed.). New York: Guilford Press.

Millon, T., Green, C., & Meagher, R. (1982). A new psychodiagnostic tool for clients in rehabilitation settings: The MBHI. *Rehabilitation Psychology, 27*, 23–35.

Millon, T., Antoni, M., Minor, S., & Grossman, S. (2006). *Millon Behavioral Medicine Diagnostic (MBMD) manual* (2nd ed.). Minneapolis, MN: Pearson Assessments.

Mills, F., Belgrave, F., & Boyer, K. (1988). Reducing avoidance of social interaction with a physically disabled person by mentioning the disability following a request for aid. *Journal of Applied Social Psychology, 14*, 1–11.

Moye, J. (1996). Theoretical frameworks for competency assessments in cognitively impaired elderly adults. *Journal of Aging Studies, 10*, 27–42.

Moye, J., Armesto, J., & Karel, M. (2005). Evaluating capacity of older adults in rehabilitation settings: Conceptual models and clinical challenges. *Rehabilitation Psychology, 50*, 207–214.

Mpofu, E., Beck, R., & Weinrach, S. G. (2004). Multicultural rehabilitation counseling: Challenges and strategies. In F. Chan, N. L. Berven, & K. R. Thomas (Eds.), *Counseling theories and techniques for rehabilitation health professionals* (pp. 386–402). New York, NY: Springer.

Mpofu, E., & Oakland, T. (Eds.). (2010). *Rehabilitation and health assessment: Applying ICF guidelines.* New York, NY: Springer Publishing.

Myerson, L. (1948). Physical disability as a social psychological problem. *Journal of Social Issues, 4*, 2–10.

Neff, W. (1971). *Rehabilitation psychology.* Washington, DC: American Psychological Association.

Nezu, A., Nezu, C., & Perri, M. (1989). *Problem-solving therapy for depression: Theory, research, and clinical guidelines.* New York, NY: Wiley.

Nosek, M. A. (2010). Women's experience of disability. In R. G. Frank, M. Rosenthal, & B. Caplan (Eds.), *Handbook of rehabilitation psychology* (2nd ed., pp. 371–378). Washington, DC: American Psychological Association.

Novack, T., Sherer, M., & Penna, S. (2010). Neuropsychological practice in rehabilitation. In R. Frank, M. Rosenthal, & B. Caplan (Eds.), *Handbook of rehabilitation psychology* (2nd ed., pp. 165–178). Washington, DC: American Psychological Association.

Nuyen, J., Spreeuwenberg, P., Groenewegen, P., Geertrudis, A., van den Bos, G., & Schellevis, F. (2008). Impact of preexisting depression on length of stay and discharge destination among patients hospitalized for acute stroke. *Stroke, 39*, 132.

Olkin, R. (1999). *What psychotherapists should know about disability.* New York, NY: Guilford.

Olkin, R. (2002). Could you hold the door for me? Including disability in diversity. *Cultural Diversity Ethnic Minority Psychology, 8*(2), 130–137.

Ortiz, S. O., & Dynda, A. M. (2010). Diversity, fairness, utility and social issues. In E. Mpofu & T. Oakland (Eds.), *Assessment in rehabilitation and health* (pp. 37–55). Upper Saddle River, NJ: Merrill.

Palmer, S., Glass, T., Palmer, J., Loo, S., & Wegener, S. (2004). Crisis intervention with individuals and their families following stroke: A model for psychosocial service during inpatient rehabilitation. *Rehabilitation Psychology, 49*, 338–343.

Parker, H. J., & Chan, F. (1990). Psychologists in rehabilitation: Preparation and experience. *Rehabilitation Psychology, 35*, 239–248.

Patterson, D., Everett, J., Bombardier, C., Questad, K., Lee, V., & Marvin, J. (1993). Psychological effects of severe burn injuries. *Psychological Bulletin, 113*, 362–378.

Patterson, D. R., & Hanson, S. (1995). Joint Division 22 and American Congress of Rehabilitation Medicine guidelines for postdoctoral training in rehabilitation psychology. *Rehabilitation Psychology, 40*, 299–310.

Patterson, D. R. (1997). Training programs in psychology. *Rehabilitation Psychology News, 24*(2), 7.

Pedersen, P. (1997). *Culture-centered counseling interventions: Striving for accuracy.* Thousand Oaks, CA: Sage.

Pegg, P. O., Jr., Auerbach, S. M., Seel, R. T., Buenaver, L. F., Kiesler, D. J., & Plybon, L. (2005). The impact of patient-centered information on patients' treatment satisfaction and outcomes in traumatic brain injury rehabilitation. *Rehabilitation Psychology, 50*, 366–374.

Perdices, M. (2005). How do you know whether your patient is getting better (or worse)? A user's guide. *Brain Impairment, 6*, 219–226.

Perdices, M., Schultz, R., Tate, R., McDonald, S., & Togher, L. (2006). The evidence base of neuropsychological rehabilitation in acquired brain impairment (ABI): How good is the research? *Brain Impairment, 7*, 119–132.

Perdices, M., & Tate, R. (2009). Single-subject designs as a tool for evidence-based clinical practice: Are they underecognised and undervalued? *Neuropsychological Rehabilitation, 19*, 904–927.

Perrin, P., Heesacker, M., Hinojosa, M., Uthe, C., & Rittman, R. (2009). Identifying at-risk, ethnically diverse stroke caregivers for counseling: A longitudinal study of mental health. *Rehabilitation Psychology, 54*, 138–149.

Peterson, D. B. (2005). International Classification of Functioning, Disability and Health: An introduction for rehabilitation psychologists. *Rehabilitation Psychology, 50*, 105–112.

Peterson, R. L., et al. (Eds.). (1992). *The core curriculum in professional psychology*. Washington, DC: American Psychological Association & National Council of Schools of Professional Psychology.

Pohjasvaara, T., Leskela, M., Vataja, R., Kalska, H., Ylikoski, R., Heitanen, M., ... Erkinjuntti, T. (2002). Poststroke depression, executive dysfunction and functional outcome. *European Journal of Neurology, 9*, 269–275.

Polite, K., & Bourg, E. (1992). Social construction of the core curriculum in professional psychology. In R. L. Peterson et al. (Eds.), *The core curriculum in professional psychology*. The National Council of Schools and Programs of Professional Psychology.

Powell, R., Johnston, M., & Johnston, D. (2007). Assessing walking limitations in stroke survivors: Are self-reports and proxy reports interchangeable? *Rehabilitation Psychology, 52*, 177–183.

Power, P. (2006). *A guide to vocational assessment* (4th ed.). Austin TX: Pro-Ed.

Prigatano, G. (1999). *Principles of cognitive rehabilitation*. New York, NY: Oxford University Press.

Prugh, D., & Eckhardt, L. (1980). Stages and phases in the response of children and adolescents to illness and injury. *Advances in Behavioral Pediatrics, 1*, 181–194.

Quale, A., & Schanke, A. (2010). Resilience in the face of coping with a severe physical injury: A study of trajectories of adjustment in a rehabilitation setting. *Rehabilitation Psychology, 55*, 12–22.

Radnitz, C., Bockian, N., & Moran, A. (2000). Assessment of psychopathology and personality in people with physical disabilities. In R. Frank & T. Elliott (Eds.), *Handbook of rehabilitation psychology* (pp. 287–310). Washington, DC: American Psychological Association.

Randolph, C. (1998). *The repeatable battery for the assessment of neuropsychological status*. San Antonio, TX: The Psychological Corporation.

Rath, J., Simon, D., Langenbahn, D., Sherr, R., & Diller, L. (2003). Group treatment of problem-solving deficits in outpatients with traumatic brain injury: A randomized outcome study. *Neuropsychological Rehabilitation, 13*, 461–488.

Rath, J., Hradil, A., Litke, D., & Diller, L. (2011). Clinical applications of problem-solving research in neuropsychological rehabilitation: Addressing the subjective experience of cognitive deficits in outpatients with acquired brain injury. *Rehabilitation Psychology, 56,* 320–328.

Reeves, M., Rafferty, A., Aranha, A., & Theisen, V. (2008). Changes in knowledge of stroke risk factors and warning signs among Michigan adults. *Cerebrovascular Diseases, 25,* 385–391.

Reid-Arndt, S., Caplan, B., Rusin, M., Slomine, B., Uomoto, J., & Frank, R. (2010). Psychological assessment and intervention in rehabilitation. In R. L. Braddom (Ed.), *Physical medicine and rehabilitation* (4th ed., pp. 65–98). Philadelphia, PA: Elsevier.

Reid-Arndt, S. A., Stucky, K., Cheak-Zamora, N., DeLeon, P. H., & Frank, R. G. (2010). Investing in our future: Unrealized opportunities for funding graduate psychology training. *Rehabilitation Psychology, 55,* 321–330.

Ricker, J. H., & Rosenthal, M. (2010). Traumatic brain injury in adults. In R. G. Frank, M. Rosenthal, & B. Caplan (Eds.), *Handbook of rehabilitation psychology* (2nd ed., pp. 43–62). Washington, DC: American Psychological Association.

Rippentrop, A. (2005). A review of the role of religion and spirituality in chronic pain populations. *Rehabilitation Psychology, 50,* 278–284.

Rivara, F., Tollefson, S., Tesh, E., & Gentilello, L. (2000). Screening trauma patients for alcohol problems: Are insurance companies barriers? *Journal of Trauma, 48,* 115–118.

Rizzo A., Schultheis, M., Kerns, K., & Mateer, C. (2004). Analysis of assets for virtual reality applications in neuropsychology. *Neuropsychological Rehabilitation, 14,* 207–239.

Roberts, M. C., Borden, K. A., Christiansen, M. D., & Lopez, S. J. (2005). Fostering a culture shift: Assessment of competence in the education and careers of professional psychologists. *Professional Psychology Research and Practice, 36*(4), 355.

Robey, R., Schultz, M., Crawford, A., & Sinner, C. (1999). Single-subject clinical outcome research: Designs, data, effect sizes, and analyses. *Aphasiology, 13,* 445–473.

Robinson, M., & O'Brien, E. (2010). Chronic pain. In R. Frank, M. Rosenthal, & B. Caplan (Eds.), *Handbook of rehabilitation psychology* (2nd ed., pp. 119–132). Washington, DC: American Psychological Association.

Robinson, R., Jorge, R., Moser, D., Acion, L., Solodkin, A., Small, S., … Arndt, S. (2008). Escitalopram and problem-solving therapy for prevention of post-stroke depression. *Journal of the American Medical Association, 299,* 2391–2400.

Rochette, A., Desrosiers, J., Bravo, G., Tribble, D., & Bourget, A. (2007). Changes in participation level after spouse's first stroke and relationship to burden and depressive symptoms. *Cerebrovascular Diseases, 24,* 255–260.

Rodolfa, E., Bent, R. J., Eisman, E., Nelson, P. D., Rehm, L., & Ritchie, P. (2005). A cube model for competency development: Implications for psychology educators and regulators. *Professional Psychology: Research and Practice, 36,* 347–354.

Rohe, D. (2010). Psychological aspects of rehabilitation. In W. Frontera (Ed.), *DeLisa's physical medicine and rehabilitation* (5th ed., pp. 387–412). Philadelphia, PA: Lippincott Williams & Wilkins.

Rose, F., Brooks, B., & Rizzo, A. (2005). Virtual reality in brain damage: A review. *CyberPsychology and Behavior, 8,* 241–262.

Rusin, M. J., & Jongsma, A. E., Jr. (2001). *The rehabilitation psychology treatment planner.* New York, NY: Wiley.

Rusin, M. J., & Uomoto, J. M. (2010). Psychotherapeutic interventions. In R. G. Frank, M. Rosenthal, & B. Caplan (Eds.), *Handbook of rehabilitation psychology* (2nd ed., pp. 259–271). Washington, DC: American Psychological Association.

Sachs-Ericsson, N., Hansen, N., & Fitzgerald, S. (2002). Benefits of assistance dogs: A review. *Rehabilitation Psychology, 47*, 251–277.

Sander, A., Witol, A., & Kreutzer, J. (1997). Alcohol use after traumatic brain injury: Concordance of patients' and relatives' reports. *Archives of Physical Medicine and Rehabilitation, 78*, 138–142.

Sbordone, R., & Long, C. (Eds.). (1996). *Ecological validity of neuropsychological testing.* Delray Beach, FL: GR Press/St. Lucie Press.

Schaefer, L. (2010). MacArthur competence assessment tools. In J. Kreutzer, J. DeLuca, & B. Caplan (Eds.). *Encyclopedia of clinical neuropsychology* (pp. 1502–1505). New York: Springer.

Schaller, J., Parker, R., & Garcia, S. B. (1998). Moving toward culturally competent rehabilitation counseling services: Issues and practices. *Journal of Applied Rehabilitation Counseling, 29*, 40–48.

Scherer, M. J., Blair, K. L., Banks, M. E., Brucker, B., Corrigan, J., & Wegener, S. (2010). Rehabilitation psychology. In I. B. Weiner & W. E. Craighead (Eds.), *The Corsini encyclopedia of psychology* (Vol. 4, pp. 1444–1447). New York, NY: John Wiley & Sons.

Schoenberger, M., Humle, F., Zeeman, P., & Teasdale, T. (2006). Patient compliance in brain injury rehabilitation in relation to awareness and cognitive and physical improvement. *Neuropsychological Rehabilitation, 16*, 561–578.

Schultheis, M., Caplan, B., Ricker, J., & Woessner, R. (2000). Fractionating the Hooper: A multiple-choice response format. *The Clinical Neuropsychologist, 14*, 196–201.

Schultheis, M., & Mourant, M. (2001). Virtual reality and driving: The road to better assessment for cognitively impaired populations. *Presence: Teleoperators and Virtual Environments, 10*, 431–439.

Schultheis, M., & Rizzo, A. (2001). The application of virtual reality technology in rehabilitation. *Rehabilitation Psychology, 46*, 296–311.

Schulz, R., Czaja, S., Lustig, A., Zdaniuk, B., Martire, L., & Perdomo, D. (2009). Improving the quality of life of caregivers of persons with spinal cord injury: A randomized controlled trial. *Rehabilitation Psychology, 54*, 1–15.

Scott, K. J., Ingram, K. M., Vitanza, S. A., & Smith, N. G. (2000). Training in supervision: A survey of current practices. *The Counseling Psychologist, 28*, 403–422.

Seale, G., Berges, I., Ottenbacher, K., & Ostir, G. (2010). Changes in positive emotion and recovery of functional status following stroke. *Rehabilitation Psychology, 55*, 33–39.

Seligman, M. E. (1998). *Learned optimism: How to change your mind and your life.* New York, NY: Vintage Books.

Seligman, M. E., & Csikszentmihalyi, M. (2000). Positive psychology: An introduction. *American Psychologist, 55*, 5–14.

Sexton, T., Hanes, C., & Kinser, J. (2010). Translating science into clinical practice. In J. Thomas & M. Hersen (Eds.), *Handbook of clinical psychology competencies* (pp. 153–182). New York, NY: Springer.

Sherer, M., Bergloff, P., Boake, C., High, W., & Levin, H. (1998). The awareness questionnaire: Factor structure and internal consistency. *Brain Injury, 12*, 63–68.

Sherer, M., Sander, A., Nick, T., High, W., Malec, J., & Rosenthal, M. (2002). Early cognitive status and productivity outcome after traumatic brain injury: Findings from the TBI Model Systems. *Archives of Physical Medicine and Rehabilitation, 83,* 183–192.

Shewchuck, R., & Elliott, T. (2000). Family caregiving in chronic illness and disability. In R. Frank & T. Elliott (Eds.), *Handbook of rehabilitation psychology* (pp. 553–564). Washington, DC: American Psychological Association.

Shontz, F. C., & Wright, B. A. (1980). The distinctiveness of rehabilitation psychology. *Professional Psychology, 11,* 919–924.

Sieh, D., Meijer, A., & Visser-Meily, J. (2010). Risk factors for stress in children after parental stroke. *Rehabilitation Psychology, 55,* 391–397.

Siller, J. (1969). Psychological situation of the disabled with spinal cord injuries. *Rehabilitation Literature, 30,* 290–296.

Sirtori, V., Corbetta, D., Moja, L., et al. (2009). Constraint induced movement therapy for upper extremities in stroke patients. *Cochrane Database System Reviews, 4,* CD004433.

Sirtori, V., Corbetta, D., Moja, L., & Gatti, R. (2010). Constraint-induced movement therapy for upper extremities in patients with stroke. *Stroke, 41,* e57–e58.

Snyder, C., Lehman, K., Kluck, B., & Monsson, Y. (2006). Hope for rehabilitation and vice versa. *Rehabilitation Psychology, 51,* 89–112.

Sohlberg, M., & Mateer, C. (2001). *Cognitive rehabilitation: An integrative neuropsychological approach.* New York, NY: Guilford Press.

Stepanski, E., Rybarczyk, B., Lopez, M., & Stevens. S. (2003). Assessment and treatment of sleep disorders in older adults: A review for rehabilitation psychologists. *Rehabilitation Psychology, 48,* 23–36.

Stein, P., Sliwinski, M., Gordon, W., & Hibbard, M. (1996). Discriminative properties of somatic and nonsomatic symptoms for poststroke depression. *The Clinical Neuropsychologist, 10,* 141–148.

Stiers W., Barisa M., Stucky K., Turner A., Pawlowski C., vanTubbergen M.,…Caplan B. (in press). Guidelines for competency development and measurement in postdoctoral training in rehabilitation psychology. *Rehabilitation Psychology.*

Stiers, W., Hanson, S., Turner, A., Stucky, K., Barisa, M., Brownsberger, M.,…Kuemmel A. (2012). Guidelines for structure and process of postdoctoral training in applied rehabilitation psychology. *Rehabilitation Psychology, 57,* 267–279.

Stoltenberg, C. D., & Grus, C. L. (2004). Defining competencies in psychology supervision: A consensus statement. *Journal of Clinical Psychology, 60,* 771–785.

Straus, S., Majumdar, S., & McAlister, F. (2002). New evidence for stroke prevention: Scientific review. *Journal of the American Medical Association, 288,* 1388–1395.

Stuss, D., Winocur, G., & Robertson, I. (Eds.). (2008). *Cognitive neurorehabilitation* (2nd ed.). New York, NY: Cambridge University Press.

Sue, D. W., & Sue, D. (2007). *Counseling the culturally diverse: Theory and practice* (5th ed.). New York, NY: Wiley.

Sullivan, M. J., Newman, R., & Abrahamson, D. J. (2007). The State Leadership Conference: A history and appreciation. *Psychological Services, 4,* 123–134.

Svoboda, E., & Richards, J. (2009). Compensating for anterograde amnesia: A new training method that capitalizes on emerging smartphone technologies. *Journal of the International Neuropsychological Society, 15,* 629–638.

Szymanski, E. (2000). Disability and vocational behavior. In R. Frank & T. Elliott (Eds.), *Handbook of rehabilitation psychology* (pp. 499–518). Washington, DC: American Psychological Association.

Tate, R. (2010). *A compendium of tests, scales and questionnaires: The practitioner's guide to measuring outcomes after acquired brain impairment.* New York, NY: Psychology Press.

Tate, R., McDonald, S., Perdices, M., Togher, L., Schultz, R., & Savage, S. (2008). Rating the methodological quality of single-subject designs and n-of-1 trials: Introducing the single-case experimental design (SCED) scale. *Neuropsychological Rehabilitation, 18,* 385–401.

Taub, E., & Uswatte, G. (2000). Constraint-induced movement therapy based on behavioral neuroscience. In R. Frank & T. Elliott (Eds.), *Handbook of rehabilitation psychology* (pp. 475–496). Washington, DC: American Psychological Association

Tedeschi, R., & Calhoun, L. (2004). Posttraumatic growth: Conceptual foundations and empirical evidence. *Psychological Inquiry, 15,* 1–18.

Temple, R., Zgaljardic, D., Yancy, S., & Jaffray, S. (2007). Crisis intervention training program: Influence on staff attitudes in a postacute residential brain injury rehabilitation setting. *Rehabilitation Psychology, 52,* 429–434.

Thomas, J. C., & Hersen, M. (2010). *Handbook of clinical psychology competencies.* New York, NY: Springer.

Thomas, K. R., & Chan, F. (2000). On becoming a rehabilitation psychologist: Many roads lead to Rome. *Rehabilitation Psychology, 45,* 65–73.

Thomas, S., & Lincoln, N. (2008). Predictors of emotional distress after stroke. *Stroke, 39,* 1240–1245.

Toedter, L., Reese, C., Berk, S., Schall, R., Hyland, D., & Dunn, D. (1995). The reliability of psychological measures in the assessment of stroke patients: Caveat inquisitor? *Archives of Physical Medicine and Rehabilitation, 76,* 719–725.

Umlauf, R., & Frank, R. (1983). A cluster-analytic description of patient subgroups in the rehabilitation setting. *Rehabilitation Psychology, 28,* 157–167.

U.S. Department of Health & Human Services. (2003). Summary of the HIPAA privacy rule. Retrieved October 28, 2010, from http://www.hhs.gov/ocr/privacy/hipaa/understanding/index.html

U.S. Department of Justice. (2005). A guide to disability rights laws. Retrieved from http://www.ada.gov/cguide.htm#anchor65610

Uswatte, G., Taub, E., Mark, V., Perkins, C., & Gauthier, L. (2010). Central nervous system plasticity and rehabilitation. In R. G. Frank, M. Rosenthal, & B. Caplan (Eds.), *Handbook of rehabilitation psychology* (2nd ed., pp. 391–406). Washington, DC: American Psychological Association.

van Wijk, I., Algra, A., van de Port, A., Bevaart, B., & Lindeman, E. (2006). Change in mobility activity in the second year after stroke in a rehabilitation population. Who is at risk for decline? *Archives of Physical Medicine and Rehabilitation, 87,* 45–50.

Vasquez, M. J. T. (2007). Cultural difference and the therapeutic alliance: An evidence-based analysis. *American Psychologist, 62,* 878–885.

Vestling, M., Tufvesson, B., & Iwarsson, S. (2003). Indicators for return to work after stroke and the importance of work for subjective well-being and life satisfaction. *Journal of Rehabilitation Medicine, 35,* 127–131.

Visser-Meily, J., Post, M., Riphagen, I., & Lindeman, E. (2004). Measures used to assess burden among caregivers of stroke patients: A review. *Clinical Rehabilitation, 18,* 601–623.

Vohs, K. D., Baumeister, R. F., Schmeichel, B. J., Twenge, J. M., Nelson, N. M., & Tice, D. M. (2008). Making choices impairs subsequent self-control: A limited resource account of decision making, self-regulation, and active initiative. *Journal of Personality and Social Psychology, 94,* 883–898.

Wade, S., & Walz, N. (2010). Family, school, and community: Their role in the rehabilitation of children. In R. Frank, M. Rosenthal, & B. Caplan (Eds.), *Handbook of rehabilitation psychology* (2nd ed., pp. 345–354). Washington, DC: American Psychological Association.

Wadley, V., McClure, L., Howard, V., Unverzagt, F., Go, R., Moy, C.,...Howard, G. (2007). Cognitive status, stroke symptom reports and modifiable risk factors among individuals with no diagnosis of stroke or transient ischemic attack in the Reasons for Geographic and Racial Differences in Stroke (REGARDS) study. *Stroke, 28,* 1143–1147.

Waldron-Perrine, B., Rapport, L., Hanks, R., Lumley, M., Meachen, S., & Hubbarth, P. (2011). Religion and spirituality in rehabilitation outcomes among individuals with traumatic brain injury. *Rehabilitation Psychology, 56,* 107–116.

Webster's Encyclopedic Unabridged Dictionary of the English Language (New Revised edition). (1996). New York, NY: Gramercy.

Wechsler, D. (2008). *Wechsler Adult Intelligence Scale, fourth edition administration and scoring manual.* San Antonio, TX: Pearson.

Wegener, S., Elliott, T., & Hagglund, K. (2000). On psychological identity and training: A reply to Thomas and Chan (2000). *Rehabilitation Psychology, 45,* 74–80.

Wegener, S., Hagglund, K., & Elliott, T. (1998). On psychological identity and training: Boulder is better for rehabilitation psychology. *Rehabilitation Psychology, 43,* 17–29.

Wegener, S., Mackenzie, E., Ephraim, P., Ehde, D., & Williams, R. (2009). Self-management improves outcomes in persons with limb loss. *Archives of Physical Medicine and Rehabilitation, 90,* 373–380.

Wegener, S., & Stiers, W. (2010). Prevention, assessment, and management of work-related disability. In R. Frank, M. Rosenthal, & B. Caplan (Eds.), *Handbook of rehabilitation psychology* (2nd ed., pp. 407–416). Washington, DC: American Psychological Association.

Wehman, P., West, M., Fry, R., Sherron, P., Groah, C., Kreutzer, J., & Sale, P. (1989). Effect of supported employment on the vocational outcomes of persons with traumatic brain injury. *Journal of Applied Behavior Analysis, 22,* 395–405.

Weinberg, J., Diller, L., Gordon, W., Gerstman, L., Lieberman, A., Lakin, P.,...Ezrachi, O. (1977). Visual scanning training effect on reading-related tasks in acquired right brain damage. *Archives of Physical Medicine and Rehabilitation, 58,* 479–486.

Wertheimer, J., Roebuck-Spencer, T., Constantinidou, F., Turkstra, L., Pavol, M., & Paul, D. (2008). Collaboration between neuropsychologists and speech-language pathologists in rehabilitation settings. *Journal of Head Trauma Rehabilitation, 23,* 273–285.

White, B., Driver, S., & Warren, A. M. (2008). Considering resilience in the rehabilitation of people with traumatic disabilities. *Rehabilitation Psychology, 53,* 9–17.

White, B., Driver, S., & Warren, A. (2010). Resilience and indicators of adjustment during rehabilitation from a spinal cord injury. *Rehabilitation Psychology, 55,* 23–32.

WHO ASSIST Working Group. (2002). The Alcohol, Smoking, and Substance involvement Screening Test (ASSIST): Development, reliability, and feasibility. *Addiction, 97,* 1183–1194.

Whyte, J., & Hart, T. (2003). It's more than a black box; it's a Russian doll: Defining rehabilitation treatments. *American Journal of Physical Medicine, 82*, 639–652.

Wilde, M. (2006). The validity of the Repeatable Battery of Neuropsychological Status in acute stroke. *Clinical Neuropsychologist, 20*, 702–715.

Williams, B. (2010). Perils of evidence-based medicine. *Perspectives in Biology and Medicine, 53*, 106–120.

Williams, L., Ghose, S., & Swindle, R. (2004). Depression and other mental health diagnoses increase mortality risk after ischemic stroke. *American Journal of Psychiatry, 161*, 1090–1095.

Williams, L. S., Kroenke, K., Bakas, T., Plue, L. D., Brizendine, E., Tu, W., et al. (2007). Care management of poststroke depression: A randomized, controlled trial. *Stroke, 38*, 998.

Wilson, B. (2002). *Neuropsychological rehabilitation.* New York, NY: Psychology Press.

Wilson, B., Emslie, H., Quirk, K., & Evans, J. (1999). George: Learning to live independently with NeuroPage. *Rehabilitation Psychology, 44*, 284–296.

Wilson, B., Herbert, A., & Shiel, A. (2003). *Behavioural approaches to neuropsychological rehabilitation.* New York, NY: Psychology Press.

Wilson, B., & Kapur, N. (2008). Memory rehabilitation for people with brain injury. In D. Stuss, G. Winocur, & I. Robertson (Eds.), *Cognitive neurorehabilitation* (2nd ed., pp. 522–540). New York, NY: Cambridge University Press.

Woessner, R., & Caplan, B. (1995). Affective disorders following mild to moderate traumatic brain injury: Interpretive hazards of the SCL-90-R. *Journal of Head Trauma Rehabilitation, 10*, 79–89.

Wolf, S., Winstein, C., Miller, J., Taub, E., Uswatte, G., Morris, D., Giuliani, C., Light, K., Nichols-Larsen, D. for the EXCITE Investigators. (2006). Effects of constraint-induced movement therapy on upper extremity function 3–9 months after stroke: The EXCITE randomized clinical trial. *Journal of the American Medical Association, 296*, 2095–2104.

Wood, S., & Kubik, J. (2005). Presenting the complex client in court: Practical issues related to the assessment of capacity. *Rehabilitation Psychology, 50*(3), 201–206.

Woodward, H., Winterbalther, K., Donders, J., Hackbarth, R., Kuldanek, A., & Sanfilippo, D. (1999). Prediction of neurobehavioral outcome 1–5 years after postpediatric traumatic head injury. *Journal of Head Trauma Rehabilitation, 14*, 351–359.

World Health Organization. (2001, May 22). *International classification of functioning, disability and health (ICF).* Geneva, Switzerland: Author.

Wortman, C. B., & Silver, R. C. (1989). The myths of coping with loss. *Journal of Consulting and Clinical Psychology, 57*, 349–357.

Wright, B. A. (Ed.). (1959). *Psychology and rehabilitation.* Washington, DC: American Psychological Association.

Wright, B. A. (1960, 1983). *Physical disability: A psychosocial approach.* New York, NY: Harper and Row.

Wright, B. A. (1993). Division of rehabilitation psychology: Roots, guiding principle, and a persistent concern. *Rehabilitation Psychology, 38*, 63–65.

Yonan, C., & Wegener, S. (2003). Assessment and management of pain in the older adult. *Rehabilitation Psychology, 28*, 4–13.

Yuker, H. E. (Ed.). (1988). *Attitudes toward persons with disabilities.* New York, NY: Springer.

Zangwill, O. L. (1947). Psychological aspects of rehabilitation in cases of brain injury. *British Journal of Psychology, 37*, 143–149.

KEY TERMS

Accommodations: Modification of environment or task parameters in the service of minimizing impact of disabilities on accessibility or task performance. Examples include making a job site wheelchair accessible, allowing extra time for task completion, providing a sign language interpreter at lectures, or using enlarged test materials. Often prefaced by "reasonable," as embodied in the Americans With Disabilities Act of 1990, which mandated such adjustments to address the needs of persons with disabilities and foster their full participation in the community.

American Board of Rehabilitation Psychology (ABRP): One of 13 specialty boards operating under the auspices of the American Board of Professional Psychology (ABPP). The ABRP is responsible for the development and maintenance of the education and training requirements and examination procedures that must be satisfied by individuals who wish to obtain ABPP board certification in rehabilitation psychology.

Americans With Disabilities Act (ADA): Federal law passed in 1990 that prohibits discrimination against persons with disabilities in vocational or educational settings unless the individual's disability prevents him or her from performing some essential function of the activity in question, even if accommodations are provided. The ADA also applies to other venues such as restaurants, public service agencies, medical facilities, and courts.

Anosognosia: Unawareness of or failure to appreciate the existence or extent of a disability such as hemiparesis or unilateral neglect. Anosognosia is most often (but not exclusively) observed in the acute phase following right hemisphere stroke. Given the neurological substrate, it is generally accepted to differ from the psychological mechanism of denial, although the two can coexist. Anosognosia can be a significant impediment to motivation for rehabilitation and can therefore hamper patient progress.

Assistive technology: Compensatory technologically oriented devices and services used by persons with disabilities, their family members, and therapists to minimize the impact of disability on particular behaviors and functions (Kirsch & Scherer, 2010). Types of devices include electronic organizers, speech synthesizers, power wheelchairs, and prismatic lenses. Services include creating new devices, modifying or repairing existing tools, and providing technical support.

Biopsychosocial Model: Paradigm in which biological, social, and psychological factors are all considered relevant in understanding individual patients. Historically, rehabilitation psychology embraced this model well before medicine or other psychological specialties, as sociocultural and environmental factors were seen as necessary elements to consider in working to enable persons with disabilities to function optimally in the community.

Capacity: The ability to make decisions with personal relevance, which requires understanding alternative choices and the likely consequences of each. Typically, the term applies to a particular ability. An individual can be determined to have one sort of capacity (e.g., to manage one's finances) but lack another (e.g., to make decisions about one's medical care).

Cognitive rehabilitation: Interventions designed to ameliorate specific cognitive deficits such as impaired attention, unilateral neglect, or executive dysfunction. Approaches have included rote repetition, training of specific compensatory strategies, computer-based practice, and virtual reality systems (Hart, 2010).

Competence: Capability of making certain decisions and/or taking certain actions. "Competence" is a legal determination by a judge and typically requires that the individual demonstrate an understanding of the issue at hand, awareness of possible options for action, grasp of the likely risks and benefits, and ability to communicate his or her choice. The term is also used in psychology to refer to an individual psychologist's demonstration of adequate capability in a specific realm of psychological practice.

Complaint-contingent medication administration: Approach to pain management in which analgesics are given when the patient voices complaints of pain. This strategy risks fostering increased complaints in order to secure pain medication.

Constraint-induced movement therapy (CIMT): Approach to motor rehabilitation in which the unimpaired (or less impaired) extremity is prevented from moving, forcing use of the affected extremity during intensive structured practice (Taub & Uswatte, 2000).

Coping: Strategies and tactics (behavioral, emotional, or cognitive) used to attempt to minimize stress by solving problems, modifying the environment, seeking support, or modulating one's emotional or physiological responses to psychologically taxing situations and events. Coping can be adaptive or maladaptive, problem focused or emotion focused.

Denial: A psychological defense mechanism whereby aspects of reality are disavowed. In rehabilitation settings, denial can present a major obstacle to progress, as patients who deny cognitive or physical deficits are unlikely to acknowledge the need for therapy and may therefore resist participating. Denial must be distinguished from anosognosia (impaired self-awareness), which is generally believed to have a neurological basis.

Disability: The result of a complex interaction between health status (usually an "impairment" as defined in the World Health Organization's International Classification of Functioning, Disability and Health (ICF) to indicate "problems in body function or structure, such as a significant deviation or loss") and environmental and/or personal factors, the result of which is restriction of an individual's ability to complete or participate in one or more fundamental activities of daily life (World Health Organization, 2001). "Disability" can also refer to an administrative decision made by an organization or regulatory agency (e.g., insurance carrier or Social Security Administration).

Diversity: Characterized by a variety of elements. "Disability" has come to be considered a "diversity feature" in rehabilitation and with respect to broad social norms on a par with race, gender, and sexual orientation (Olkin, 2002).

Division 22: The Division of Rehabilitation Psychology of the American Psychological Association that is primarily concerned with matters of disability and chronic illness and their prevention and treatment.

Ecological validity: Predictive validity of a test for daily life functioning, a critical feature of psychological assessment in rehabilitation settings (Marcotte & Grant, 2010).

Function: As conceptualized in the World Health Organization's ICF, this term has multiple meanings. It can refer to the activity of an organ or body part, to a daily life activity such as cooking or driving, or to the individual's participation in society.

Handicap: Inability or diminished ability to execute one or more essential activities of daily living due to a personal (e.g., paralysis) or environmental obstacle (e.g., steps leading to entrance to a building). In the ICF scheme, "handicap" is a frequent, but not invariable, corollary of "disability."

Health Insurance Portability and Accountability Act (HIPAA): Federal law that regulates access to and use of protected health information (PHI) by designated covered entities. PHI is patient information that is unique to that individual and provides clues to or would allow identification of the individual. The law was designed to foster patient confidentiality, to promote the use of electronic health records (which dictated rules limiting access to patient information), and to prevent individuals from losing health insurance because of a change in residence or employer. Rehabilitation psychologists, especially those working in team settings, must balance their obligations to confidentiality under HIPAA with their responsibilities to the treating team.

Impairment: Limitation or deficit/decline in usual functioning. In the World Health Organization's ICF scheme, "impairments" are considered to be manifestations of dysfunction of bodily structure or function and are distinguished from any underlying disease or disorder.

Individuals With Disabilities Education Act (IDEA): Federal legislation that provides funding for special education. Services provided under IDEA must be offered in the "least restrictive environment."

Interdisciplinary team: The common modus operandi in rehabilitation in which treatment is delivered by professionals from several disciplines, typically physical medicine, physical therapy, occupational therapy, speech pathology, rehabilitation nursing, and rehabilitation psychology (Butt & Caplan, 2010). Recreational therapists, nutritionists, social workers, and case managers may also be team members. In contrast to the "multidisciplinary team," there is some overlap in roles and functions of different team members.

International Classification of Functioning, Disability and Health (ICF): Model of disability proposed by the World Health Organization (2001). An earlier version employed "disabling" language (e.g., "impairment," "handicap") and designated the locus of disability in the individual, whereas the ICF is couched in more neutral terminology and emphasizes the impact of the person's environment on his or her participation in society.

Multicultural competence: Awareness of the various "individual difference" factors noted previously under "diversity" and ability to take these into account when providing clinical services or conducting research.

Multidisciplinary team: Group of individuals of varying professional backgrounds and expertise who collaborate for purposes of patient care. This team model differs from the "interdisciplinary team" model in that roles and responsibilities generally do not cross professional boundaries.

Nonstandard assessment: Related to "testing the limits" during assessment, nonstandard approaches involve modifications of test items or administration procedures that aim to eliminate or minimize the impact of construct-irrelevant factors. Examples include displaying visual stimuli in a column rather than horizontally to reduce the effect of unilateral neglect and offering multiple choices for persons with expressive language problems. Nonstandard assessment may also involve creation of novel tests to allow finer-grained assessment of component cognitive processes (e.g., Caplan & Caffery, 1992).

Person-first language: Terminology concerning persons with disabilities in which the disability itself is placed last—for example, "person with a traumatic brain injury" instead of "brain-injured person." A corollary concerns "nondisabling language," for example, referring to a "stroke survivor" rather than "stroke victim."

PLISSIT model: Acronym representing a phased approach to sexual counseling consisting of the following steps: giving **P**ermission (legitimizing the topic), providing **L**imited **I**nformation, offering **S**pecific **S**uggestions, and **I**ntensive **T**herapy (Annon, 1974).

Quality of life: The degree to which an individual derives satisfaction from life. A multiply determined phenomenon encompassing psychological, physical, familial, social, vocational, and environmental factors. Enhanced quality of life is historically a fundamental goal of rehabilitation.

Rehabilitation Act of 1973: A forerunner of the Americans With Disabilities Act, legislation that guaranteed certain rights to people with disabilities. In particular, Section 504 forbids discrimination by employers, organizations, or other groups on the basis of disability. Individuals with disabilities cannot be denied services or opportunities to participate because of their disability.

Rehabilitation psychology: The psychological specialty concerned with congenital or acquired conditions causing physical and/or mental disabilities and chronic illness, their effects on the individual and significant others, and intervention methods (Scherer, Blair, Banks, Brucker, Corrigan, & Wegener, 2010). Rehabilitation psychologists work—often as part of a treatment team—to promote optimal physical, psychological, and interpersonal functioning.

Requirement of mourning: A tenet of early conceptualizations of "adjustment to disability" and "stage theories" of adjustment according to which it was imperative that an individual with an acquired disability (e.g., spinal cord injury) go through a period of grieving the losses (physical, vocational, social, etc.) caused by their disability before they could become "adjusted." This notion is no longer widely accepted.

Resilience: Behavioral and/or emotional flexibility in adapting to stressful experiences. A key concept in the field of positive psychology and one that is congruent with rehabilitation's historical emphasis on "ability, not disability." Craig (2012) defined the term with reference to people with disabilities as "…the process of maintaining stable psychological, social, and physical functioning when adjusting to the effects of a physical disability and subsequent impairment."

Self-awareness: Understanding of one's strengths, weaknesses, emotional states, and environment. Diminished self-awareness often accompanies conditions such as stroke or traumatic brain injury that are commonly treated in rehabilitation settings and can sabotage motivation for therapy.

Stage theory: The notion—now largely discredited—that an individual's response to a stressful event (such as new-onset disability) consists of a set series of emotional responses through which the individual passes in sequence, eventually (ideally) reaching the final stage of "adjustment" to his or her disability.

Time-contingent medication administration: Method of pain management in which analgesics are administered at regular intervals rather than in response to patient report of pain. This approach is felt to foster reduced pain behavior, as medication is not administered in response to pain complaints.

Transdisciplinary team: Model of collaborative patient care in which there is significant overlap across disciplinary boundaries.

INDEX

Academy of Rehabilitation Psychology, 8
Adjustment to disability
    family, 65–66, 88, 129–32
    patient, 63–65, 86–88, 112–16, 129–32
Administration, management, 143–48
Advocacy, 93–94, 101–6
Alcohol use/abuse, 77–78, 95, 140–41
Alcohol Use Disorders
    Identification Test, 78
American Board of Clinical
    Neuropsychology, 63
American Board of Professional
    Psychology (ABPP), 7–8, 53–54
American Board of Rehabilitation
    Psychology (ABRP), 7, 41, 42,
    50, 53–54, 86, 101, 109, 143
American Psychological Association
    (APA), 41, 50–51. *see also*
    APA Ethics Code
Americans With Disabilities Act
    (ADA), 27–28, 67–69, 91, 101–3
Amputations, 4, 94, 95, 115, 120–22
Anderson, C., 131, 134–35
Animals, service, 98
Anosognosia, 108, 130, 133
Antidepressants, 130, 134–35
Anxiety
    adjustment to disability, 129
    assessment, consultation, 93, 94
    interventions, 108, 112–16, 122, 134
    patient resilience, 129
    social factors impact on, 137
APA Ethics Code
    advertising, public statements, 21
    assessment, 23–24
    bartering, 22

beneficence and nonmaleficence, 17
competency, 19–20, 34–35, 53
confidentiality, privacy, 18, 21, 28–29
discrimination, 35
diversity, 34–35
education, training, 22
enforceability, 34
ethical issues, resolving, 19
ethical standards, 18–25
fidelity and responsibility, 17
general principles, 17–18
harassment, 35, 46–47
human relations, 20, 35, 42, 44–45
information requests, 24
informed consent, 23, 24, 35
integrity, 17–18
justice, 18
overview, 16–17
record keeping, fees, 21–22
research and publication, 22–23
respect for rights and dignity, 18, 34, 42
sexual intimacy, 25, 46
supervision, 144
testimonials, 21
treatments, therapy, 23–25
violations, reporting, 19
APA Multicultural Guidelines, 33–39
Arango-Lasprilla, J., 139–40
Arnold, N., 116
Artman, L. K., 38, 102
Asians, 37
Assessment
    adjustment to disability (family),
    65–66, 88, 129–32
    adjustment to disability (patient),
    63–65, 86–88, 112–16, 129–32

180 Index

Assessment (*Cont.*)
  APA Ethics Code, 23–24
  aptitude measurement tools, 68
  board certification, 59, 63
  capability *vs.* performance, 67
  cognitive abilities, 71–73, 89–90
  consultation (*see* Consultation)
  decision-making capacity, 74–76
  depression, 65–69, 79, 89–96
  educational/vocational
    capacities, 67–69, 90–91
  emotional functioning, 69–71
  empirical research, 132–33
  extent/nature of disability,
    identification of, 66–67
  function emphasis, 62–63
  memory (*see* Memory)
  nature and history of, 60–62
  neuropsychological, 62–63, 67–68,
    71–73
  pain, 76–77, 91–92, 116–17
  personality, emotional
    status, 69–71, 93–94
  physical functioning, 96–97
  preserved abilities, 66–67
  process, 59–60
  risk taking behaviors, 70, 77–78
  self-reports, 133
  sexual functioning, 73–74, 95–96
  social, behavioral functioning, 78–79
  substance use/abuse, 77–78, 95, 140–41
  terminology choices, 73
  testing *vs.*, 61–62
  tools, 132–33
  translation of interpretations,
    61, 64–65, 70, 72–73, 93–94
Assistive technology, 97–98, 118–19, 136
ASSIST questionnaire, 78
Association membership, 53, 105–6
Association of State and Provincial
  Psychology Boards (ASPPB), 25
Attitude, 48
Avoidant coping, 133
Awareness of self and others, 43–44.
  see also self-awareness
Awareness Questionnaire, 133

Backhaus, S., 134
Baltimore Conference on Rehabilitation
  Psychology Postdoctoral Training, 10
Banos, J., 139
Barisa, M., 128
Barnett, S., 126
Barrett, A., 119, 136
Bartolucci, A., 131
Batten, S., 133
Baumeister, R.F., 90
Beedie, A., 115
Behavior
  cognitive-behavioral therapy, 115–16, 134
  functioning, 86–88
  modification, 116–18, 138
Behnke, S. H., 28
Ben-Yishay, Y., 119
Berges, I., 130
Bernard, J. M., 143–44
Berninger, V., 72
Berry, J., 70, 131
Biofeedback, 118
Boake, C., 139
Board certification
  assessment, 59, 63
  consumer protection, 101–6
  professional identity, 50, 53–54
Bockian, N., 70
Bombardier, C., 78, 95
Boundaries, 45–46
Bourg, E., 48
Bowman, M., 139
Braga, L., 135
Brain injury. *see* traumatic
  brain injury (TBI)
BrainSTARS, 91
Brenner, L. A., 9
Brief Symptom Inventory (BSI), 70
Brucker, B., 7–8
Bruyère, S. M., 102–3
Burns, 52, 63, 84, 94, 120–22
Bush, S., 30
Butt, L., 82, 104

CAGE questionnaire, 78
Calhoun, L., 132

Callahan, C. D., 103–4, 128
Capacity (legal), 30, 53, 74–76, 104
Caplan, B., 7–8, 23, 68, 72, 82, 85, 104, 113
Caregivers
  adjustment of, 114–16, 129–32
  assessment, 84
  depression in, 139–40
  social support, 131
Cerebral palsy, 4, 52, 72, 118
Certification. *see* board certification
Chan, F., 50, 125
Cheak-Zamora, N., 103
Chen, Y., 138
Christopher, M. S., 32
Chwalisz, K., 125
Cicerone, K., 135–36
Clark University Conference, 5
Clock drawing, 72
Code, C., 127
Cognitive-behavioral therapy, 115–16, 134
Cognitive functioning, 71–73, 89–90
Cognitive rehabilitation, 118–20, 135–36
Commission for Accreditation of
    Rehabilitation Facilities (CARF), 7
Compensatory skill building, 121–22
Competency
  APA Ethics Code, 19–20, 34–35, 53
  legal status, 30, 53, 74–76, 104
Computers, 98, 136
Confidentiality
  APA Ethics Code, 18, 21, 28–29
  interpersonal interactions, 47
Connors, T., 72
Constraint-induced movement
    therapy (CIMT), 118
Consultation
  advocacy, 93–94, 101–6
  agent role, 99
  anxiety (*see* anxiety)
  in assessment, 61
  assistive technology, 97–98, 118–19, 136
  behavioral functioning, 86–88
  bodily disfigurement, 94
  cognitive functioning, 71–73, 89–90
  communication, 85
  consultant, expectations/roles, 82–85, 99

cultural, language concerns, 88–89
definitions, 81
educational/vocational
    capacities, 67–69, 90–91
interventions, 120–21
laws, 93–94, 101–6 (*see also*
    ethics and legal issues)
life-planning report, 92
mental health framework, 85
pain, 76–77, 91–92, 116–17
personality, emotional
    status, 69–71, 93–94
physical functioning, 96–97
referrals, 84, 85
resources, 91
sexual functioning, 73–74, 95–96
substance use/abuse, 77–78, 95, 140–41
team approach, 82, 111
treatment models, 82
treatment noncompliance, 86–88
Consumer protection, 101–6
Continuing education, 53
Cook, C., 132
*Core Curriculum in Professional
    Psychology*, 47
Counseling, 114–16, 131
Cox, D. R., 7–8, 51, 52
Cox, R., 7–8
Crowe, S., 132
Culture. *see also* diversity
  competency, 32–39
  consultation, 88–89
  disability, perceptions of, 38, 136–37
  interpersonal interactions, 44
  multicultural variables, defining, 37–39

Daniels, J. A., 38, 102
Davis, L., 131
Decision-making capacity, 74–76
DeLeon, P. H., 103
Dembo, T., 3
Dementias, 52, 84
Department of Veterans
    Affairs, 3, 9, 75–76
DePaz, A., 135
De Piano, F., 60–61

Depression
  adjustment to disability, 129–32
  antidepressants, 130, 134–35
  assessment, 65–69, 79, 89–96
  behavioral modification, 86–88
  in caregivers, 139–40
  cognitive-behavioral therapy, 115–16, 134
  inpatient treatment, 122
  interventions, 108, 111–16, 122, 134
  patient resilience, 129
  post stroke, 131, 134–35
  prevention, 137–38
  social support, 131
  stage theory, 64, 130
Diagnostic and Statistical Manual of Mental Disorders, 61, 111
Diller, L., 66, 134
Disability
  adaptive value change, 39
  adjustment to (*see* adjustment to disability)
  concepts of, 37–38
  determinations, 29
  meaning, finding, 39
  as minority status, 38
  posttraumatic growth, 132
  social psychology of, 38, 136–37
Diversity. *see also* culture
  APA Ethics Code, 34–35
  APA Multicultural Guidelines, 33–39
  case vignettes, 33
  cultural competency, 32–39
  defined, 33–34
  gender differences, 37–38
  multicultural variables, defining, 37–39
  overview, 31–33
  research, 139–40
Division 22 Newsletter, 6
Doleys, D., 77
Dreer, L., 131
Driver, S., 129
Duff, J., 115
Dunn, D., 137
Dunn, M., 121, 137

Eckhardt, L., 113
Education. *see* training
Educational/vocational
  capacities, 67–69, 90–91
Ehde, D., 115
Electronic communication, 47
Elliott, T., 64, 69, 70, 131, 138
Emotional functioning, 69–71
Empathy, 43
Engel, G. L., 5
Ephraim, P., 115
Eskes, G., 119
Ethical Principles of Psychologists and Code of Conduct. *see* APA Ethics Code
Ethics and legal issues
  Americans With Disabilities Act (ADA), 27–28, 67–69, 91, 101–3
  APA Ethics Code (*see* APA Ethics Code)
  capacity, 30, 74–76, 104
  children, education of, 26–27
  competency, 30, 53, 74–76, 104
  consultation, 93–94
  disability determinations, 29
  Family Education Rights and Privacy Act (FERPA) of 1974, 27
  Family Medical Leave Act, 69
  Health Insurance Portability and Accountability Act (HIPAA), 28–29
  Individuals With Disabilities Education Act (IDEA), 26–27, 102
  interpersonal interactions (*see* Interpersonal interactions)
  interventions, withholding, 127
  overview, 15–16, 25, 30
  person-first language, 29, 38
  reasonable accommodations, 26, 69, 91, 93, 103
  Rehabilitation Act of 1973, 26
  resources, 25
  Social Security Disability Insurance (SSDI), 29
  Uniform Guardianship and Protective Proceedings Act of 2009, 75
Evans, M., 115
Exercise, 117

Falender, C. A., 145
Family Education Rights and Privacy Act (FERPA) of 1974, 27

Family Medical Leave Act, 69
Fann, J., 126
Feintuch, U., 136
Fields, A. J., 33
Financial concerns, 46
Follette, R., 128–29
Fordyce, W. E., 91, 116
Foundation for Rehabilitation
 Psychology, 6
Frank, R. G., 103
Frankl, V. E., 39
Freeman, K., 128
Functional Assessment
 Measure (FAM), 139
Functional Independence
 Measure (FIM), 138–39

Gans, B., 72
Gans, J., 121
Garcia, S. B., 37
Garrett, J., 4
Garro, L. C., 32–33
Giger, J., 131
Glass, T., 131, 135
Glueckauf, R. L., 39, 51
Gold, S., 60–61
Goodyear, R. K., 143–44
Grant, J., 131
Green, B., 139
Grus, C. L., 144, 145
Guilmette, T., 73
Gusman, F. D., 39

Hackett, M., 131, 134–35
Hall, K., 139
*Handbook of Clinical Psychology
 Competencies*, 112
Hanes, C., 125
Hanks, R., 139
Hanson, S., 24, 28, 30, 52
Harassment, 35, 46–47
Hart, T., 126
Hatcher, R. L., 51
Heinemann, A., 62
Heinrich, R., 70
Hemiplegia, 4, 72, 118
Hess, D. W., 7

Hibbard, M. R., 7, 52, 112
Hicken, B., 138
HIPAA, 28–29
Hooper Visual Organization Test, 72
Hoskin, K., 132
House, A., 134–35
Hradil, A., 134

Ibarra, S., 134
Identity, professional. *see*
 Professional identity
Individuals With Disabilities Education
 Act (IDEA), 26–27, 102
Informed consent, 23, 24, 35
International Classification of
 Functioning, Disability and
 Health (ICF), 103, 110
Internships, 51, 145, 146
Interpersonal interactions
 attitude, 48
 awareness of self and others, 43–44
 boundaries, 45–46
 concepts of, 41–42
 confidentiality, privacy, 47
 educational, training program
  standards, 47–48
 electronic communication, 47
 empathy, 43
 ethics in, 42 (*see also* Ethics
  and legal issues)
 family of patient, 88
 financial concerns, 46
 harassment, 35, 46–47
 human relations, 44–45
 multicultural factors, 44
 professionalism, 45–46
 sexual behavior, 46
 stress, 45
 supervision, 143–48
 sympathy, 43
Interventions
 ABCs of, 112
 adjustment, 63–65, 86–88, 112–16
 advocacy, 104
 APA Ethics Code, 23–25
 assessment (*see* Assessment)
 assistive technology, 97–98, 118–19, 136

Interventions (*Cont.*)
  avoidant coping, 133
  behavior modification, 116–18, 138
  biofeedback, 118
  challenges in, 108, 127
  cognitive-behavioral therapy, 115–16, 134
  cognitive rehabilitation, 118–20, 135–36
  compensatory skill building, 121–22
  competency, 112
  conceptualizations of, 109–12
  constraint-induced movement therapy (CIMT), 118
  consultation, 120–21 (*see also* Consultation)
  counseling, 114–16, 131
  crisis approach, 135
  definitions, 107
  depression (*see* Depression)
  empirical research, 134–36
  family, consideration of, 135
  inpatient psychologist's role, 108, 121–22
  motivational interviewing, 117, 138
  outpatient psychologist's role, 108–9
  patient resilience, 114
  patients involved in, 107–8
  positive psychology, 63, 114
  problem-solving therapy, 130–31, 134–35
  resources, 111–12
  sexual function, 117–18
  social skills training, 121
  stroke, 20, 51
  targets, goals, 110–11
  team approach, 82, 111
  team-attended psychological interview (TAPI), 121
  terminology, 110
  treatment models, 82
  treatment noncompliance, 86–88
  treatment plans, 111–12, 134
  virtual reality (VR) technology, 119, 136
  withholding, 127
Ipsen, C., 116

Jackson, H., 132
Jacobson, N., 128–29
Jaffray, S., 135
Jongsma, A. E., Jr., 111–12, 134

Kaslow, N. J., 145
Katz, N., 136
Keany, K., 39
Kennedy, P., 115
Kerkhoff, T., 24, 28, 30, 33
Kerns, K., 136
Kinser, J., 125
Kirsch, N., 97–98, 136
Kizony, R., 136
Klyce, D., 134
Kortte, K., 133
Kubik, J., 104
Kurylo, M., 138

Ladany, N., 145
Lakes, K., 32–33
Langenbahn, D., 134
Language
  consultation, 88–89
  person-first, 29, 38
La Roche, M., 32
Larson, P. C., 3, 6, 7
Latinos, 33, 37
Layman, D. E., 7, 112
Leahy, M., 68, 69
Lee, D., 139
Legal issues. *see* Ethics and legal issues
Lehrman-Waterman, D., 145
Levin, H., 135–36
Leviton, G., 3
Lewin, K., 125
Lewis, B. L., 51
Life-planning report, 92
Lifetime Practice Excellence Award, 8
Lim, M., 128
Lincoln, N., 131
Lindeman, E., 131
Linley, P., 132
Litke, D., 134
LoGalbo, A., 139
Lollar, D., 103
Loo, S., 131, 135
Lopez, S. R., 32–33

Mackenzie, E., 115
Malec, J., 130, 134, 135–36
Mallinson, T., 62

Mateer, C., 136
McDonald, S., 127
McGrath, J., 132
McMillen, J., 132
Mehta, S., 134
Memory
   assessment, 63, 67–68, 71, 89
   assistive technology, 98
   consultation, 89
   interventions, 108, 111, 115, 118
   self-generation strategies, 135–36
Mentors, 44, 54–55, 146
Meyerson, L., 3, 5
Millis, S., 139
Moessner, A., 130
Money Management Survey (MMS), 132
Moran, A., 70
Motivational interviewing, 117, 138
Mpofu, E., 38, 103
Multiple sclerosis, 71, 95, 124–26
Myerson, L., 137

National Council of Schools and Programs in Professional Psychology (NCSPP), 48, 107
National Council on Psychological Aspects of Disability (NCPAD), 6
National Council on Psychological Aspects of Physical Disability (NCPAPD), 6, 41, 42
Native Americans, 37
Naveh, Y., 136
Neurorehabilitation, 6
Niemeier, J., 139–40
Nosek, M. A., 37
Novack, T., 84, 124, 126, 139

Oakland, T., 103
O'Keefe, J., 102–3
Olkin, R., 38
Ostir, G., 130
Ottenbacher, K., 130

Pain
   assessment, 76–77, 91–92, 116–17
   behaviors, 116–17
Palmer, J., 131, 135

Palmer, S., 131, 135
Parker, H. J., 7–8, 50
Parker, R., 37
Pate, W. E., 51
Patterson, D. R., 52
Pedersen, P., 36
Pegg, P. O., Jr., 115, 134
Penna, S., 84, 124
Perdices, M., 127, 128
Personal digital assistants (PDAs), 98, 118, 136
Personality, emotional status assessment, 69–71, 93–94
Person-first language, 29, 38
Physical disability: A psychological approach (Wright), 4
Physical functioning assessment, 96–97
PLISSIT model, 96, 118
Polite, K., 48
Politics, 104–5
Positive psychology, 63, 114
Post, M., 131
Posttraumatic growth, 132
Power, P., 68
Pressure sores, 138, 140
Prevention, 137–38
Prigatano, G., 119
Princeton Conference, 4, 5
Privacy. *see* Confidentiality
Problem-solving therapy, 130–31, 134–35
Professional identity
   association membership, 53, 105–6
   board certification, 50, 53–54
   components, 50
   concepts of, 49
   continuing education, 53
   education, training, 50–52
   mentoring, 44, 54–55
   specialty, areas of focus within, 52–53
Professionalism, 45–46
Prugh, D., 113
Psychological Practices With the Physically Disabled (Garrett & Levine), 4
Psychology and Rehabilitation (Wright), 4

Quadriplegia, 64, 72
Quale, A., 114

Radnitz, C., 70
Raimy, V., 4
Randomized controlled trial
    (RCT), 126–28
Rath, J., 134
Raven Coloured Progressive Matrices, 72
Ravesloot, C., 116
Reasonable accommodations,
    26, 69, 91, 93, 103
Rehabilitation Act of 1973, 26
Rehabilitation psychology
    Baltimore Conference on Rehabilitation
        Psychology Postdoctoral Training, 10
    Clark University Conference, 5
    concepts of, 4–5, 10–11
    Division of Rehabilitation Psychology
        (APA Division 22) evolution, 5–7
    early roots of, 3
    future trends, 9–10
    Princeton Conference, 4, 5
    publications, early, 3–4
    Rehabilitation Psychology XXXX, 8–9
    research (see research)
    specialty certification
        establishment, 5, 7–8
    terminology, 110
    theoretical roots of, 62
    training (see training)
Rehabilitation Psychology (journal),
    5, 9, 63, 103, 125, 130
Rehabilitation Psychology (Neff), 4
Rehabilitation Psychology
    Conference, 8–9
Reid-Arndt, S. A., 60, 74, 103
Relationships, rapport. see
    Interpersonal interactions
Reliable change index, 128–29
Religion, spirituality, 38, 69–70, 113, 140
Repeatable Battery for the Assessment
    of Neuropsychological
    Status (RBANS), 132
Research
    assessment (see Assessment)
    barriers in rehabilitation
        settings, 126–27
    development of, 123–25

diversity (see Diversity)
evidence base, 129
interventions (see Interventions)
outcomes, 138–39
posttraumatic growth, 132
prevention, 137–38
randomized controlled
    trial (RCT), 126–28
reliable change index, 128–29
single-subject designs (SSDs), 127–29
substance use/abuse, 77–78, 95, 140–41
Resilience, 114, 129. see also
    Adjustment to disability
Revenstorff, D., 128–29
Ricci, A., 7–8
Ricker, J., 72, 139
Ring, H., 136
Riphagen, I., 131
Risk taking behaviors, 70, 77–78
Rivera, P., 70, 131
Rizzo A., 136
Rodolfa, E., 53
Rohe, D., 7–8, 78
Rosenthal, M., 7–8
Rusin, M. J., 108, 111–12, 134

Sachs, P. R., 3, 6, 7
Schaller, J., 37
Schanke, A., 114
Scherer, M. J., 10, 97–98, 136
Schultheis, M., 72, 136
Schultz, R., 127
Seale, G., 130
Seekins, T., 116
Self-awareness
    anosognosia, 108, 130, 133
    awareness of self and others, 43–44
    promotion of, 44, 48, 130
Sexton, T., 125
Sexual behavior, 46
Sexual function, 73–74, 95–96, 117–18
Sexual intimacy, 25, 46
Shechter, J., 23, 68, 113
Sherer, M., 84, 124, 139
Sherr, R., 134
Shewchuck, R., 131

Shontz, F. C., 7
Simon, D., 134
Single-subject designs (SSDs), 127–29
Sleep disorders, 87
Smart phones, 118, 136
Social, behavioral functioning
 assessment, 78–79
Social Security Disability
 Insurance (SSDI), 29
Social skills training, 121
Speech deficits, 72, 89–90
Spinal cord injury
 adjustment to, 113–15, 131
 as area of focus, 52–53, 63
 assessment, 66, 69–71, 73–74, 77
 behavior modification, 117
 cognitive-behavioral therapy, 115–16, 134
 consultation, 84
 depression (see Depression)
 ethics and legal issues, 34–35
 pressure sores, 138, 140
 sexual functioning, 73–74, 95–96
 substance use/abuse, 77–78, 95, 140–41
 treatment, 20, 121–22
St. James, P., 72
Stewart, R. K., Jr., 7, 112
Stoltenberg, C. D., 144
Stress, 45
Stroke
 adjustment to, 113, 129–32
 antidepressants, 130, 134–35
 as area of focus, 52–53
 assessment, 63, 66, 71–74, 79
 behavior modification, 117
 cognitive-behavioral therapy, 115–16, 134
 complications, management of, 110
 consultation, 84
 depression (see Depression)
 prevention, 137–38
 sexual functioning, 73–74, 95–96
 social support, 131
 treatment, 20, 51
 treatment noncompliance, 87
Stucky, K., 103
Stuss, D., 135–36
Substance use/abuse, 77–78, 95, 140–41

Sue, D. W., 37
Supervision, 143–48
Sympathy, 43
Symptom Checklist-90-Revised, 70
Szymanski, E., 68

Tate, R., 127, 128, 138
TBI. *see* Traumatic brain injury (TBI)
Team approach, interventions, 82, 111
Team-attended psychological
 interview (TAPI), 121
Tedeschi, R., 132
Temple, R., 135
Terrio, H., 9
Thomas, S., 131
Togher, L., 127
Trail Making Test, 72
Training
 accreditation, 51
 APA Ethics Code, 22
 behaviors, modeling, 146
 case vignettes, 33
 clinical experiences, 51
 competency, 143–48
 continuing education, 53
 history of, 7, 8, 10
 internships, 51, 145, 146
 interpersonal interactions
  standards, 47–48
 mentors, 44, 54–55, 146
 postdoctoral programs, 52
 practicum, 51
 professional identity, 50–52
 supervision, 143–48
Traumatic brain injury (TBI)
 adjustment to, 113–15, 130, 131
 as area of focus, 52–53
 assessment, 70, 71, 74, 77, 89
 behavior modification, 117
 children, 91
 cognitive rehabilitation, 118–20, 135–36
 consultation, 84, 87–89
 educational/consultation programs, 91
 informed consent, 35
 motivational interviewing, 117, 138
 outcome measures, 139

Traumatic brain injury (TBI) (*Cont.*)
  perceived self-efficacy, 134
  person-first language, 29, 38
  problem-solving therapy, 130–31, 134–35
  sexual functioning, 73–74, 95–96
  substance use/abuse, 77–78, 95, 140–41
  training in, 20, 51
  treatment, present-day, 20, 33, 51, 121–22, 134
  treatment historically, 6
Treatment. *see* Interventions
Treatment plans, 111–12, 134
Trexler, L., 134
Turner, A., 78, 95

Umlauf, R., 64, 70
Uniform Guardianship and Protective Proceedings Act of 2009, 75
Uomoto, J. M., 108

Vanderploeg, R. D., 9
Vasquez, M. J. T., 33
Veiel, L., 133
Virtual reality (VR) technology, 119, 136
Visser-Meily, J., 131
Visual impairment, 72

Vocational/educational capacities, 67–69, 90–91
Vocational rehabilitation, 3, 68

Wadley, V., 137–38
Waldron-Perrine, B., 140
Warren, A. M., 129
Wechsler scales, 72–73
Wegener, S., 115, 131, 133, 135
Weiss, P., 136
Whelan, J., 7–8
White, B., 129
Whyte, J., 126, 135–36
Wilde, M., 132
Williams, B., 127
Williams, R., 115
Willmuth, M., 7–8
Wilson, B., 136
Woessner, R., 72
Wood, S., 104
Wright, B. A., 3, 4, 7, 31–32, 36, 38, 101–3, 110

Yancy, S., 135
Ylvisaker, M., 135

Zgaljardic, D., 135

ABOUT THE AUTHORS

David R. Cox, PhD, ABPP, is Executive Officer of the American Board of Professional Psychology. He is board certified in Rehabilitation Psychology by the American Board of Professional Psychology and was a founding member of the American Board of Rehabilitation Psychology. He is President of Neuropsychology & Rehabilitation Consultants, P.C., in Chapel Hill, North Carolina. Dr. Cox has served on the staff and faculty of U.C. San Diego, Duke University, the University of North Carolina at Chapel Hill, and the University of Florida. He is a Fellow of the American Psychological Association (Divisions 22 and 42) and a Fellow of the National Academy of Neuropsychology. He is a recipient of the Heiser Award of the American Psychological Association and Lifetime Practice Excellence Award from APA Division 22. He is a past president of the Florida Psychological Association and recipient of that organization's Distinguished Practitioner Award, Distinguished Service Award, and Legislative Affairs and Public Policy Board Chapter Representative of the Year. His work has extended to national levels, as he has served on various committees and task forces within professional psychology including the APA Taxonomy Work Group and the Council of Credentialing Organizations in Professional Psychology; he has also served on workgroups and committees with the Department of Defense and Defense Health Board and was the lead consultant in establishing a multidisciplinary team of rehabilitation, neuropsychology, and computer experts with IBM for development of one of the first cognitive rehabilitation computer programs, the IBM THINKable System®. He has helped establish community re-entry programs for persons with brain injury and also established the Neuropsychology Department (now Medical Psychology Department) of Florida Hospital. He has widely presented and published in the areas of rehabilitation, neuropsychology, and competency in professional psychology.

Richard H. Cox, MD, PhD, DMin, ABPP, is Adjunct Professor, Psychiatry and Behavioral Sciences, Duke University Medical School; Research Scholar, Center for Clinical BioEthics, Georgetown University Medical School; Affiliate Fellow, Potomac Institute, Washington, DC; and Emeritus President/Professor, Forest Institute of Professional Psychology. Dr. Cox has served on the faculty of Northwestern University Medical School and Rush University Medical School and is a Member of the Oxford Roundtable, Oxford University (UK). He has served as consultant to numerous national and international health service organizations including the World Health Organization and United Nations. Dr. Cox was a member of the founding team and was the founding President of the American Board of Rehabilitation Psychology. He is board certified in both Rehabilitation Psychology and Clinical Psychology and is Diplomate in Marriage and Family Therapy, Pastoral Counseling, and Clinical Hypnosis, the American Academy of Family Physicians, and the American Academy of Pain Management. He serves on the Editorial Board for PsycCritiques. Dr. Cox has received numerous awards including the Distinguished Service Award, Division 22; and the Jefferson Silver Cup, the Heiser Award, the President's Citation for Distinguished Service, and the Lifetime Achievement Award—all from the American Psychological Association. He has been awarded three honorary doctorates (DSc, PsyD, DHL) for his professional services in the United States and third world countries. Dr. Cox has served on numerous American Psychological Association committees, presented at annual meetings, and published 19 chapters in books, over 75 journal articles, and 14 books.

Bruce Caplan, PhD, ABPP, FACRM, is board certified in both Rehabilitation Psychology and Clinical Neuropsychology by the American Board of Professional Psychology and is a Fellow of the American Psychological Association, National Academy of Neuropsychology, and American Congress of Rehabilitation Medicine. Dr. Caplan serves as Senior Editor of *Journal of Head Trauma Rehabilitation* and is a member of the editorial boards of *Topics in Stroke Rehabilitation* and *Rehabilitation Psychology*. He previously served as Editor of *Rehabilitation Psychology*. In 1987, Dr. Caplan edited the first comprehensive rehabilitation psychology textbook (*Rehabilitation Psychology Desk Reference*), and he was Coeditor of the four-volume *Encyclopedia of Clinical Neuropsychology*. He is Past President of the Philadelphia Neuropsychology Society and of Division 22 (Rehabilitation Psychology) of the American Psychological Association. He is the recipient of two Distinguished Service Awards and the Lifetime

Achievement Award from Division 22. Dr. Caplan was a founding member of the American Board of Rehabilitation Psychology. Currently in independent practice, he was formerly Professor and Chief Psychologist in the Department of Rehabilitation Medicine at Jefferson Medical College.

ABOUT THE SERIES EDITORS

Arthur M. Nezu, PhD, ABPP, is Professor of Psychology, Medicine, and Public Health at Drexel University and Special Professor of Forensic Mental Health and Psychiatry at the University at Nottingham in the United Kingdom. He is a Fellow of multiple professional associations including the American Psychological Association, and board certified by the American Board of Professional Psychology in Cognitive and Behavioral Psychology, Clinical Psychology, and Clinical Health Psychology. Dr. Nezu is widely published, is incoming Editor of the *Journal of Consulting and Clinical Psychology*, and has maintained a practice for three decades.

Christine Maguth Nezu, PhD, ABPP, is Professor of Psychology and Medicine at Drexel University and Special Professor of Forensic Mental Health and Psychiatry at the University at Nottingham in the United Kingdom. With over 25 years of experience in clinical private practice, consultation/liaison, research, and teaching, Dr. Maguth Nezu is board certified by the American Board of Professional Psychology (ABPP) in Cognitive and Behavioral Psychology and Clinical Psychology. She is also a Past President of the ABPP. Her research has been supported by federal, private, and state-funded agencies, and she has served as a grant reviewer for the National Institutes of Health.